HONESTLY GLUTEN FREE & DAIRY FREE

Recipes, Tips and Solutions for the Home Cook

Written & Photographed by
Sarah Stout, ND, CCN

ISBN: 150292949X
ISBN 13: 9781502929495
Library of Congress Control Number: 2014919020
CreateSpace Independent Publishing Platform
North Charleston, South Carolina

This cookbook is dedicated to my family and friends. I would like to extend and extra special thanks to my parents for sampling my recipes, even when they did not turn out as planned. I am overwhelmingly thankful for my loving mother and dear sister who reviewed and edited my book. I am infinitely grateful for my precious baby boys and my beloved husband Mike, who has graciously tested recipes, good and bad, and sacrificed extensive hours of time while I worked all hours of the day and night. I love you so very much!

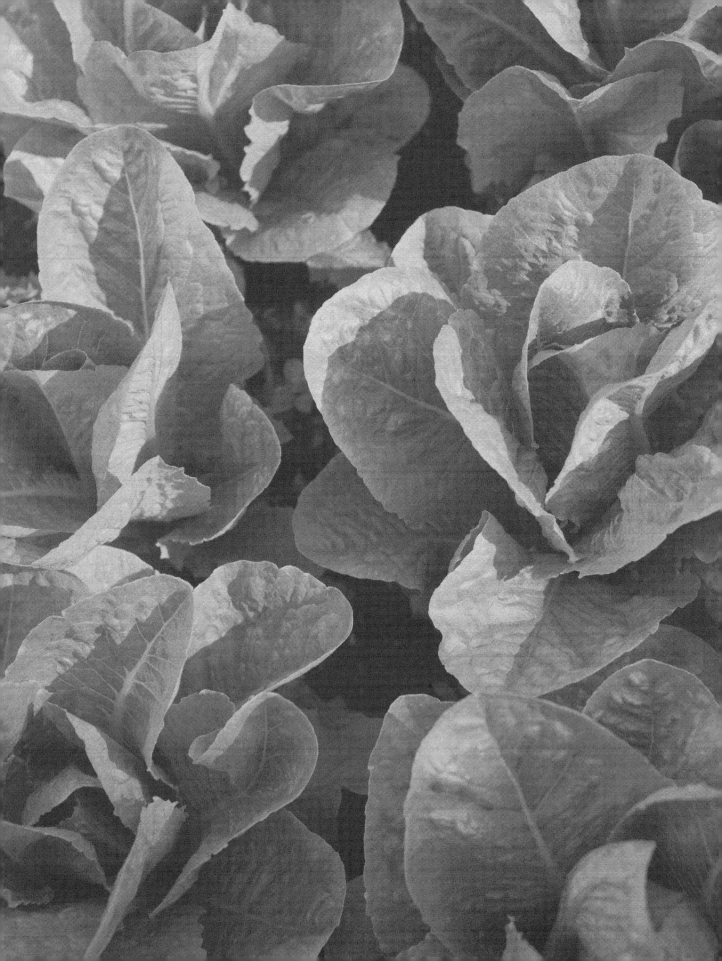

TABLE OF CONTENTS

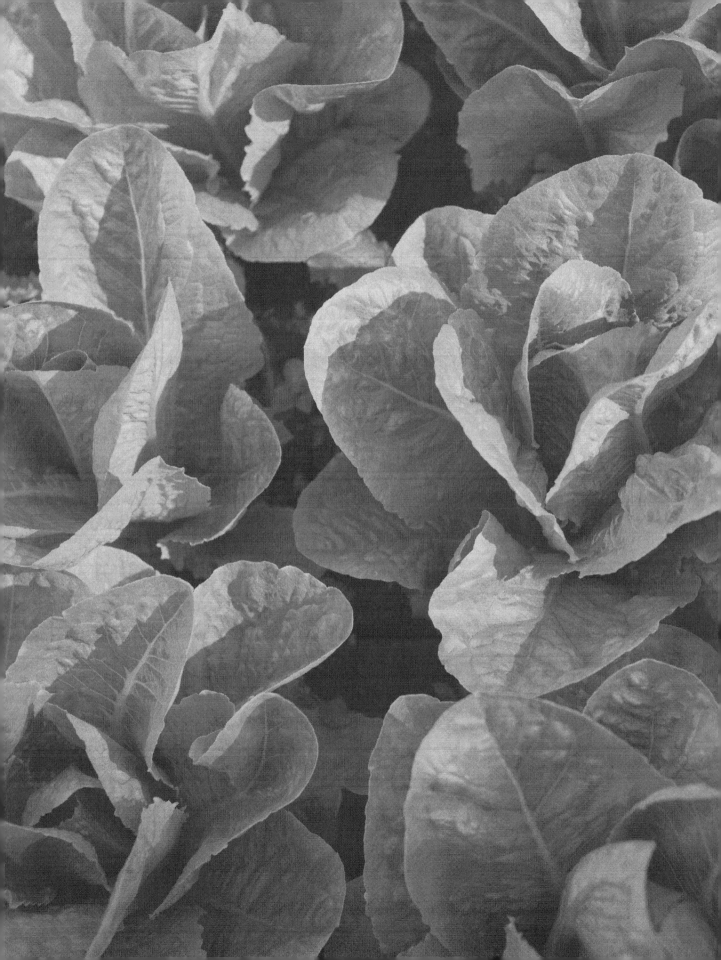

PREFACE

I have been interested in fitness, health, and wellness since I was a child. I was athletic and loved to eat fruits and vegetables. Unfortunately, I also loved sweets, refined carbohydrates, dairy products, and soda. Although I once believed my childhood generally was healthy, I came to realize my memories included multiple infections several times a year, from bronchitis to sinus infections to "twenty-four-hour" viruses. I woke up every morning in my teens extremely groggy, with stiff joints and a bloated stomach. My hair was dry, there were dark circles under my eyes, and my skin had a yellow tinge. I often felt depressed or anxious and would find lighting, loud restaurants, and smoky rooms distracting. I also found that some foods really caused me gastric distress. Once I got to college, my diet was anything but pristine, and I found myself sleeping often throughout the day. I thought it was due to late nights as a bartender but now realize it was likely caused by the foods I ate that were poison to my body—wheat bread, cheese, ice cream, frozen yogurt, liquor, and other sweet treats.

In my midtwenties I started to experience numerous health issues, and, therefore, when I began my journey toward my naturopathy and nutrition career, it was for selfish reasons. Although I have always been a healthy weight, had normal blood pressure, and exercised daily, my cholesterol was high, my energy was low, I suffered from hypothyroidism, I battled psoriasis, and my digestive tract was a total mess. I also lost hair by the handful, stopped menstruating, and experienced migraines and sinus issues regularly. Then I got mononucleosis. My body was trying to tell me something, and I didn't understand that my immune system had shut down. As a result, I developed several food allergies, as well as a terrible *Candida* infestation, and became infertile.

I attempted to seek help from several doctors, but few could help, and many were not even willing to listen to my concerns and instead offered anti-anxiety medications. Many professionals suggested seeking out a psychiatrist who could prescribe stronger medication. In a desperate effort, I tried any prescription offered, from antifungals to steroids, to handle my ailments, but my health continued to decline. I even did intravenous chelation and was told it would heal me. Instead, I became weaker, lost fifteen pounds on my already underweight frame, and felt worse than ever. That was the moment I became determined to get back my health by taking matters into my own hands. I enrolled in nutrition school, read every alternative medicine article and book I could get my hands on, took nursing classes, enrolled in naturopathy school, and discovered the connections between strong immunity, inflammation control, and good health. I realized that the childhood years of eating a poor, nutrient-deficient diet; using chemical-laden cleaners, hygiene products, and cosmetics; and being exposed to secondhand smoke when I had tended bar in college had severely impacted my overall health. I began with changing my lifestyle and modifying my diet, and miracles began to happen.

The most difficult part was abandoning familiar foods that had been a large part of my childhood, because not only did they taste good to me, but they also were part of my memories. How could I bear to give up my favorite treats and meals forever? Were they affecting my health? How would I celebrate successes without treating myself to my fondest foods? What helped me through the emotional, physical, and spiritual struggle was recognizing that making permanent changes guaranteed me a future—a healthy future. After just a few short months, my cravings for the foods I had been missing the most, such as breads, sweets, and gooey cheese, dissipated. I now follow a predominately vegetarian gluten-, soy-, egg-, and dairy free diet. I also avoid all genetically modified foods (GMOs) such as corn, sugar, and machine-made foods. My lifestyle experienced a huge transition, but now I cannot even fathom including these items in my diet. The few times I have been cross contaminated, I found that the foods no longer met my needs and were often unpalatable. For example, just a few cheese shreds taste like mold to me. Chewing gum has a metallic taste, and processed foods all have a chemical and unappealing aftertaste.

PREFACE

As you can see, although my journey was not easy, it was all worth it. I have restored my livelihood and health. I recently had a baby, which proves that the body is miraculous and can heal itself through simple yet meaningful changes in diet and lifestyle. I sincerely hope this book will be an invaluable guide to support you in your journey to optimal health and wellness. I am excited for you and the years of true life and vibrancy awaiting you!

Bon Appetit!
XOXO, Sarah

INTRODUCTION

We all want to feel good, look good, and be happy. We live in a world where taking prescription or over-the-counter (OTC) drugs is "normal," environmental pollution is prominent, and autoimmune diseases have afflicted over twenty three million Americans (Health, 2012). An autoimmune disease occurs when the body's immune system mistakenly begins to attack healthy tissue and cells. Although the actual cause of this abnormal response is not understood, there are several known triggers for autoimmune disease such as viruses, bacteria, parasites and toxins. It also can stem from family history or unhealthy lifestyle habits such as smoking or chronic stress (Committee, N.S., 2005). It seems that true health is never within reach for any of us. Many people express concern about their future, yet it seems our society is more concerned with the fuel we put in our cars than the fuel we ingest for our bodies. We are exposed daily to hundreds of food advertisements offering good health, more satiety, quicker weight loss, and extreme flavor. Yet Americans continue to get heavier and unhealthier each day as a result of eating these so-called health foods.

It is scary to think that most of the food products carried in grocery stores today are not foods at all. They are man- or machine-made products that are oversaturated with chemicals, additives, food dyes, genetically modified organisms (GMOs), highly refined starches and sugars, and, often, heavy metals which are individual metals that negatively affect health. These "foods" do not provide the nourishment nature intended for human consumption. Gone are the days of visiting our home garden or roadside produce stand to pick fresh vegetables for dinner that night or raising our own chickens and eggs for consumption. The food products offered in the inner aisles at the grocery store have changed drastically over the past few decades due to the ability to produce lower-quality crops in a more efficient manner through the use of cutting-edge technology. However, our bodies have not evolved to accept chemicals as nourishment. Therefore, we must make sense of the fact that if we want to live a healthy and abundant life, we must turn to the proper fuel for our body—whole foods, primarily plant-based whole foods.

It is no surprise that cancer rates have skyrocketed even though technological improvements have been made to successfully beat cancer. I am confident that it is because we continue to fill our bodies with harmful chemicals and carcinogenic substances we apply on our skin and ingest through our food on a daily basis. The foods we have traditionally consumed have become specialty items available only at a high price or have been replaced by highly processed food items made with cheaper ingredients. Our bodies do not recognize these foods and instead either discard or store the substances as fat. Because there are few nutrients in the foods themselves, we subject ourselves to malnutrition. Not only is the food we consume changing how our genes are expressed (University of Massachusetts Medical School, 2013), but it is also leading to chronic diseases, autoimmune disorders, chronic inflammation, and allergies. And we are becoming a very overweight yet undernourished society as a whole.

Based on my experience, changing one's diet and lifestyle makes a significant impact on overall health, longevity, youthfulness, and mental health. As Hippocrates stated, "Food is our medicine." The body is complex, but it is not complicated. The body craves simplicity, and if we provide the body nourishment from whole foods, it can heal itself. The solution to your health ailments lies in your hands. Are you ready for your life to begin?

WHAT FOODS ARE BEST FOR ME?

WHOLE FOODS

Whole foods are foods that are unprocessed and unrefined. In other words, whole foods are consumed in the same state as or minimally processed from what was harvested by Mother Nature. Whole foods are generally unaltered by man, with their nutrients still in highly available forms. Some examples of whole foods include raw fish, unpasteurized eggs, raw fruits and vegetables, unhulled grains, and unshelled nuts and seeds.

Raw foods, when consumed fresh, contain a perfect blend of vitamins, minerals, nutrients, and enzymes. Raw foods are whole foods. Raw foods are also living foods. By consuming foods in the raw form, there is a greater likelihood that you will absorb a higher ratio of nutrients than when consumed in cooked form. The cooking process can leach a portion of the essential nutrients from the food by destroying the natural enzymes that help humans break down and assimilate the food. Cooking or dehydrating food at temperatures less than 115 degrees Fahrenheit helps maintain the nutrients and enzymes. It is important to note, however, that those with compromised gastrointestinal systems should refrain from incorporating too many raw foods as once because it can worsen symptoms. A raw food diet is not for everyone.

When a food is processed and refined, the food may lose many of its beneficial properties and can even gain negative or unwanted substances, including chemicals, metals, and other toxic residues and contaminants. For example, whole grains contain three layers in each grain. The outer and most inner layers contain the most fiber and nutrients while the middle layer is very low in nutrients. In processing, the outer and inner layers are removed leaving only the middle layer. As a result, food manufacturers often add nutrients such as fiber and fillers to the grain for sale (Bauer, n.d.). In some cases, almost two-thirds of the nutrients can be lost in the food manufacturing process (Minnesota

Department of Health, n.d.). The additives contribute to the demise of one's health because they are difficult for the body to process and often are stored in the body for long periods of time, especially in those individuals who are already at risk for disease. A strict raw food diet is not suitable for everyone however adding fresh fruits and vegetables is beneficial in most circumstances.

When a diet includes processed foods, the body often becomes malnourished and overridden with toxin residues. Food manufacturers are required to replace only five nutrients (niacin, riboflavin, thiamin, folic acid and iron) lost in the refining process even though over thirty nutrients are lost (Lehman, 2015). The problem is that the nutrients added are not in the most readily available forms, are chemical based, and are at times of no use to the body. In some cases a diet high in refined foods can actually deplete the body of essential nutrients necessary for proper human growth and function, leading to poor health. When a body is malnourished, it will hold on to excess weight because it will think it is starving regardless of how many calories are consumed. This is because the body stores energy to use as a resource in times of famine. Unfortunately, our society is laden with individuals who are extremely malnourished but are morbidly obese. My clients who weigh the most eat the least. Although the human body is designed to handle stress and toxins, there is a maximum threshold. If unhealthy foods are consumed on occasion, the body will rebound from the circumstance and rid the body of the toxins accordingly; however, the body performs optimally when the unhealthy foods are avoided. Organic foods, particularly animal products and produce, also are best to purchase because pesticide and other chemical residues on foods do have a direct impact on the health of the body. Organic foods also taste more delicious and have a lengthy shelf life if stored properly. The best way to ensure you are getting the freshest and most vital produce is to eat seasonally.

EATING SEASONALLY

Eating seasonally ensures you are getting the freshest and best produce available. When eating these fresh foods, you will find that the flavors are much more pleasing to the palate, just like the experience of biting into an apple picked fresh off the apple tree. When produce is consumed in the freshest form, it is also the most nutritious, as the enzymes are still intact and the nutrients have not decomposed. The longer the time from when a vegetable or fruit is harvested to consumption, the more the nutrients break down, resulting in a lower density of essential vitamins and nutrients, which also depletes flavor.

For a complete listing of those produce items in season for your geographical area, log onto www.cuesa.org.

UNPROCESSED FOODS

Unprocessed foods include those food items that:

- Contain no artificial or man-made ingredients
- Are not manipulated in the packaging process through the addition of ingredients, preservatives or other substances (i.e. bag of baby spinach versus a box of creamed spinach)
- Contain only whole food ingredients
- Do not undergo any type of refinement process
- Do not pose a health risk when consumed in reasonable quantities
- May not have a nutritional panel

Unprocessed food is any food that can be prepared at home using ingredients from scratch or grown in a garden. In other words, think to yourself, "How did my great-grandmother prepare food?"

HOW DO I BECOME "UNPROCESSED"?

- Replace premade sauces with added sugars or other additives with fresh, homemade sauces.
- Do not consume canned fruits or vegetables. Frozen varieties are acceptable.
- Replace sugar with raw honey, date paste, or maple syrup, which fall under the whole food category, unlike processed sugars.
- Make your own juices and unsweetened fruit sauces.
- Use only whole grains like hulled brown rice, quinoa, or millet.
- Choose to eat foods only in their original form, as nature intended.

The easiest road to success is to take some time, perhaps two to three months, to be clear about your intentions and set your guidelines. Ask yourself if you will you be 100 percent compliant, or are you simply trying to make an attempt to eat better and cut out as much refinement as possible? What are your boundaries, and what are your barriers to success?

Do What Works for You!

1. **Implement changes one at a time, until you get used to them.** It may take a year, but you will continue to eat as healthy as possible.

2. **Focus 100 percent on the desired change, one step at a time.** Don't deviate!

3. **Take moderate steps, if needed, but do not use them as an excuse.** For example, instead of cutting out donuts, cut out all baked sweets. Too small steps make things too easy.

4. **Always replace unhealthy foods with the healthy foods you enjoy**. If you don't like beets, work your way up to them and instead focus on the healthy foods you do like.

What are the benefits of a pure and simple lifestyle?

Switching to an unprocessed lifestyle has extensive health benefits:

- Immune system is stronger
- Energy levels improve
- Toxins are flushed from the body daily
- Whole foods provide a positive effect on the spirit
- Increased nutrient absorption and assimilation
- Anti-aging benefits
- Dietary fiber consumption increases while sugar consumption decreases
- Inflammation is drastically reduced
- Weight management is easier and more natural
- Positive environment and community effects as well

What foods are readily available in nature?

- Seasonal produce
- Legumes, nuts, and seeds
- Food from natural animal sources
- Pure and sanitary water

When preparing your meals, I strongly suggest filling your plate at least half full with vegetables, and always include some type of leafy green such as spinach, Swiss chard, kale, arugula, or collard greens. You then should continue filling the plate with healthy, whole foods, including beans, gluten free whole grains, and animal protein if desired. My meal plate usually includes a medium tossed salad with various colorful veggies, one-quarter cup whole grains, and one-half cup legumes. I also include some items that enhance the salad experience such as nutritional yeast, hempseeds, pumpkin seeds, or nut cheese. Make certain that your salad is beautiful and colorful and then you will want to eat it! Eating with your eyes is so important and will keep you satisfied longer. Colorful food equals pure enjoyment!

Produce

- Ripe avocados
- Fresh dates (Medjool or Bahri are my favorites)
- Fresh herbs: basil, cilantro, thyme, oregano, garlic, parsley, dill, lavender fronds, and chives
- Ripe bananas: great for freezing to make ice cream
- Salad mix
- Portobello and shiitake mushrooms
- Fresh ginger
- Carrots
- Beets
- Sprouts
- Peppers
- Onions

- Thai young coconuts
- Tomatoes
- Sweet potatoes
- Greens: spinach, swiss chard, collards, turnip greens, kale, arugula, watercress
- Seasonal produce
- Jicama
- Garlic
- Celery
- Cucumber
- Broccoli
- Cauliflower
- Radishes
- Summer and winter squash varieties: zucchini, yellow crooked neck, spaghetti squash, butternut, acorn, kabocha and other winter varieties
- Fresh fruit: apples, bananas, pears, peaches, mangoes, papaya, pineapple, berries, cherries, lemons, limes, oranges, grapefruit, etc.

PANTRY RAID

Now that you've read how the foods you consume affect your overall health and vitality, the best way to get started with your healthy lifestyle is to remove all foods that do not serve your body's highest good right from the start. You can begin by removing all white foods from your pantry, including white rice, flour, sugar, and white potatoes. You should also rid your pantry of anything that has more than five ingredients on the ingredients label or that is allergenic for you or your family members. Meals and food items that come in a can, box, or bag, have no place in your pantry. Instead, stock your pantry with healthful, nutrient-dense foods that promote optimal health and vitality.

Items that I keep in stock in my pantry include:

- **Grains:** brown rice, red rice, wild rice, millet, quinoa, gluten free oat groats, teff, and sorghum. You also could choose to stock buckwheat and amaranth. Additionally, although somewhat processed, you may choose to have transitional grain foods such as cream of rice, cream of buckwheat, grits, polenta, and gluten free noodles in your pantry.

- **Beans:** dry and canned adzuki, great northern, cannellini, garbanzo, black, kidney, pinto, red, navy, cranberry, and lima beans, lentils (in all varieties), split peas, black eyed peas.

- **Sea vegetables (seaweed products):** nori (roasted seaweed) sheets, dulse flakes, kombu or wakame, hijiki. These can be found at health foods stores or in Asian markets.

- **Condiments:** coconut aminos, organic Dijon mustard, organic balsamic vinegar, raw organic apple cider vinegar, gluten free red wine vinegar, sriracha sauce, hot sauce, gluten free tamari, canned coconut milk, nutritional yeast, gluten free Worcestershire sauce.

- **Seeds and nuts:** pumpkin seeds, sunflower seeds, hempseeds, poppy seeds, sesame seeds, chia seeds, apricot kernels, walnuts, pecans, almonds, cashews, hazelnuts, pine nuts, macadamia nuts, brazil nuts, etc.

- **Spices:** Celtic sea salt, pink Himalayan salt, bay leaves, garam masala, curry powder, cumin, chili powder, coriander, turmeric, oregano, thyme, basil, fennel seed, mustard seed, cayenne pepper, black pepper, cinnamon, ginger, nutmeg, sage, garlic powder, onion powder, sumac, natural flavoring extracts such as orange or lemon oil and organic vanilla extract.

- **Misc:** powdered and canned coconut milk, organic stock, organic tomato paste in a tube (for easy access and storage), grade B maple syrup, yacon syrup, coconut palm sugar, coconut nectar, pure leaf stevia, raw honey, lucuma powder, raw cacao powder, carob powder, mesquite flour, shredded coconut, unflavored vegan gelatin, organic psyllium powder, Hain Feather Lite Baking Powder, Ener-G baking soda substitute or traditional baking soda, organic cornstarch, pharmaceutical-grade vegan protein powder, sundried tomatoes, dried mushrooms, liquid smoke, chili paste or sambal

- **Dried fruits:** dates, figs, unsulfured apricots, fruit juice sweetened cherries, cranberries, and blueberries, goji berries, raisins, shredded unsweetened coconut

- **Spreads:** unsweetened apple butter, fruit juice sweetened jam, raw almond butter, sunflower seed butter, coconut butter, other raw nut or seed butters as desired

- **Oils:** extra virgin coconut oil, extra virgin olive oil, avocado oil, pumpkin seed oil, walnut oil, grapeseed oil, sesame oil, rice bran oil

- **Beverages:** kombucha tea bags, herbal and green teas, high-quality coconut water, Teechino Dandelion Tea, matcha tea
- **Snacks:** organic brown rice and/or corn, falafel, or hummus chips; Guiltless Gourmet organic corn tortilla chips; 80 percent or greater soy free dark chocolate such as Viviani, Theo, Chocolate Decadence, or Equal Exchange brands; organic popping corn; INBars, Candice Bars, MacroBars or homemade bars

Remember to try to buy organic, and if you cannot find it in your local store, consider purchasing online. Often you can find the same products for less!

UNPROCESSED POWER FOODS TO ENERGIZE THE BODY

Power foods are those that are rich in nutrient concentration and boost the ability of the body to handle stress. Power foods boost the immune system, facilitate the natural cleansing process of the body, and enhance energy production throughout the body. They also help regulate mood, emotion, and appetite. Power foods are a wonderful addition to the diet because they provide remarkable nutrition to help increase overall health and well-being. My favorite power foods include:

- **Goji berries:** extremely rich source of iron and B vitamins, help increase longevity, have anti-aging properties; although a nightshade, inflammation is generally minimal, and Goji berries are also wonderful for female hormone balance.
- **Maca:** adaptogen that is rich in protein and contains high levels of amino acids, helps increase energy and vitality and is known for balancing the hormones and sex organs.
- **Baobab powder:** extremely rich in vitamin C, iron, calcium, and potassium, and it is wonderful for boosting immunity, aiding in digestion, and perhaps preventing cancers.
- **Lucuma:** a dried fruit powder from Peru that has a caramel-like flavor and is a good source of potassium, calcium, and magnesium; it has been linked to increased athletic performance and contributes to a strong immune system.
- **Hempseed:** wonderful source of vegetarian protein that is easy to assimilate and digest; good source of omega-3 fatty acids and vitamin E.

- **Spirulina:** fantastic source of protein and trace minerals and helps alkalize the body.
- **Asian mushrooms:** strong cancer-fighting properties, good source of vitamin D, helps the body adapt to stress.
- **Dulse, nori, and other sea vegetables:** natural source of iodine and helps chelate harmful metals from the body; beneficial in cases of adrenal fatigue, hormone dysfunction, and cholesterol regulation.
- **Cacao:** extreme source of magnesium and copper, increases dopamine production, regulates mood, decreases risk of heart attack, and increases energy; raw cacao does contain caffeine, and some brands test high in cadmium, so it is recommended to use occasionally.
- **Nutritional Yeast:** inactive yeast used in cooking. It is candida friendly and has a cheese-like flavor. It does not leaven and is extremely rich in B vitamins including vitamin B12 which is generally found in animal-based protein, and it contains all eighteen amino acids.
- **Mesquite:** made from ground pods from the mesquite tree found in dry desert-like areas; high in protein, calcium, magnesium, iron, and zinc; has a rich flavor that is a cross between brown sugar, cocoa powder, and cinnamon with hints of caramel—this is one of my favorite power foods to put in smoothies or bake into cookies.

PANTRY NECESSITIES FOR TRADITIONAL RECIPES

Below are items that I keep in my pantry at all times so I can continue to make my own minimally processed baked goods and breads at home. Although these aren't considered to be "pure", they do allow you to bake traditional recipes when the desire arises.

Baking powder: Baking powder is a leavening agent used in baked goods to provide rise. It increases the volume and lightens up baked goods, providing puffiness and airiness. It can be used instead of yeast in some baked goods when combined with fermented or acidic foods like apple cider vinegar or lemon juice. Hain makes a sodium-free baking powder that I love. Be certain to purchase aluminum- and corn-free varieties.

Baking soda: Baking soda is a leavening agent (sodium bicarbonate) used in baked goods to provide rise and spread. Products using baking soda should be baked immediately in order to prevent collapse. Ener-G makes a baking soda substitute for those watching sodium intake.

Extracts and flavorings: These include vanilla, maple, lemon, almond, and others. I recommend purchasing alcohol-free varieties, if available. Also be certain to buy gluten free extracts as some contain barley or other malt products that are not gluten free.

TIPS FOR PREPARING HEALTHY YET DELICIOUS MEALS

- Season food with herbs and spices or lemon or lime juice in lieu of condiments and sauces.
- Incorporate beans into your diet daily, rotating the types daily or weekly.
- Eat healthy plant-based fats, such as avocados, extra virgin olive oil, nuts, or seeds, daily.
- Start your day with a smoothie that contains mostly greens and small amounts of fruit.
- Increase the nutrition of soups and chilies by serving over a bed of greens or adding shredded vegetables like carrots, kale, zucchini, or jicama and adding seaweed to increase mineral content.
- Buy nuts and seeds in bulk packages (not from bins as they potentially can be cross-contaminated from surrounding bins, using contaminated scoops, etc.) They are also more likely to lose freshness quickly if not stored properly so it is best to place them in an airtight container set on the counter for easy, quick, and healthy snacking.
- Do a wet sauté by using water or vegetable broth for cooking instead of oil.
- Cook grains such as gluten free oatmeal, rice, or quinoa in bulk, freezing in individual portions for reheating at a later time.
- Eat veggies in the morning for a fresh start to your day (smoothie, omelet, or just sautéed in avocado oil or vegetable broth).
- Bake with whole grain or nut flours only. Keep starchy flours to a minimum as they are not nutritious, even though they help create a desirable mouth feel.

WHAT FOODS ARE BEST FOR ME?

- Avoid artificial or processed sweeteners (high fructose corn syrup, sucralose, sorbitol…), dyes (Red #5, Yellow #6…), additives (gum arabic, carrageenan…), preservatives (sorbates, nitrates…), and fillers (bulking agents and starches) at all times.
- Exchange sweets for fresh fruit or fruit sauces topped with a few teaspoons of chopped or melted vegan eighty percent or more dark chocolate.
- Roast veggies twice a week, being certain to incorporate at least one new vegetable and rotating according to season.
- When eating a fattier meal, always start with a large, fresh green salad and drink sixteen ounces of purified water within two hours of completing your meal.
- If you eat meat, I recommend eating only wild fish, grass fed meats, and farm-fresh eggs to ensure maximum nutrition and optimal taste.
- Make your own salsa, guacamole, and hummus to avoid unnecessary preservatives.
- Top salads and grain dishes with seeds, roasted chickpeas, or crushed organic gluten free crackers instead of croutons.
- Avoid premade salad dressings—make your own or use lemon juice, salsa, guacamole, cider vinegar, or thinned hummus for a better and tastier dressing.
- Puree beans into sauces, like pasta sauce, for added fiber and protein.
- Read labels, and avoid any food that has any ingredients you do not recognize.

OPTIMIZING HEALTH THROUGH HEALTHY HABITS

LONGEVITY

In order to maximize health, well-being, and longevity, it is important to note that we truly are what we eat. All foods have energy, and the fresher the food, the greater the energetic intensity present in the food. When food is exposed to high cooking temperatures or oxygen, it can lose some of its nutrient content (Self Nutrition Data, n.d.). Foods rich in antioxidants penetrate every cell of our bodies when consumed, allowing free radicals (damaged cells) such as those that cause cancer to be destroyed, new cells to regenerate, and tissues and muscles to be restored and rebuilt (Ipatenco, 2014). Therefore understanding that food, like people, has energy and life, helps us understand that the quality and quantity of food does matter. It only makes sense that a fresh head of organically grown cabbage picked from the garden this morning will have a fresher taste and texture than canned cabbage. If we leave the head of cabbage in the fridge for an extended period of time, it will decay and die. Therefore, the best way to maximize your quality of life and longevity is to eat fresh, seasonal foods and to avoid dead, processed foods. This does not mean you have to become a raw food enthusiast or green juice addict (although green juices can be highly nutritious and healing to the body); however it will require making conscious decisions when choosing your meals. By maximizing the amount of alkaline, natural foods in your diet, the less likely premature aging or cellular degradation will result. I experienced wonderful changes in my skin when I began to eat in this manner. Cellulite is minimized, energy is maximized, wrinkles begin to fade, and gray hair disappears (McCluskey, 2012) (Dannie, 2014). Really!

UNDERSTANDING CRAVINGS

Cravings are the body's natural mechanism to signal that it is depleted of energy and essential nutrients critical for it to carry on its functions. Cravings could mean the body is deficient in particular vitamins and minerals and is asking you to refill its reserve. It is important to note that a craving does not mean you can eat whatever you want. For example, if you are hankering for a slice of German chocolate cake, it does not mean your body is deficient in cake. It may be an indication of deficiency in an essential mineral, such as copper or magnesium, which are both found in chocolate.

Cravings also can be a result of emotional dissatisfaction. For instance, around the holidays we spend more time with friends and family and sometimes reminisce about family traditions and pleasant childhood memories. If you find yourself craving your grandmother's warm tapioca pudding, it is not likely that you are lacking the nutrients found in the pudding, but you may be longing for the loving touch or companionship of your grandmother. It is important for you to tap into your craving to determine if you really hungry or if are you merely bored, sad, or lonely. Why are you eating?

Sometimes the body will crave the foods that are the most harmful for it, as is often the case with gluten and dairy allergies and intolerances. In fact, gluten and dairy contain morphine-like chemicals within the molecular structures themselves which act as a neurotoxin on the brain. As a result, the brain sends signals for you to eat more and more of the food, even though it is causing harm to your body and its DNA cells. The chemical in gluten is called gluteomorphin and in dairy it is casomorphin. Years after giving up dairy and gluten, I still test positive for antibodies to these chemicals, which helps me understand why I could never imagine giving up cheese and crusty breads. I have to admit it was difficult at times, but the longer I abstained, the easier it became to resist temptation. In fact, I now find cheesy and bready foods to be completely unappealing (from the girl who once loved fresh Italian bread and cheesecake).

LIFESTYLE CHANGES WITH REGARD TO FOOD CHOICES

Inflammation

Inflammation is the body's immediate first-aid reaction to heal itself from damage caused by a virus, a bacteria, a fungus, an environmental toxin, or an injury. This is how the body restores itself (Sears, 2005).

Phases of Inflammation

- **Acute:** The body responds to damage by immediately repairing the damage. Symptoms can be mild or unnoticeable.
- **Chronic:** The body has to continuously fight off a repeat offender, such as, for instance, food intolerances, *Candida*, *H. pylori*, or heavy metal toxicity. The body becomes weakened over time due to stress. A way to assess chronic inflammation is to have a physician test your C-reactive protein (CRP) which is used to assess heart disease, stroke risk and shows the potential for other diseases (Healthwise Staff, 2014).

Once the immune system is compromised, all forms of chronic disease can occur. These include, but are not limited to, the following:

- Diabetes
- Weight issues
- Cancer
- Heart disease
- Stroke
- Alzheimer's disease
- Parkinson's disease
- Fibromyalgia
- Multiple sclerosis
- Rheumatoid arthritis
- Lupus
- Degenerative disorders
- Food allergies/intolerances/sensitivities

The key to optimal health is to prevent your body from entering the state of chronic inflammation.

The truth is there is NO MAGIC PILL for chronic inflammation.

Culprits of chronic inflammation (American Heart Association, 2015) include the following:

- Fungi such as *Candida*
- Bacteria, including but not limited to *H. pylori* (responsible for peptic ulcers) and *Borrelia burgdorferi* (responsible for Lyme disease)
- Viruses such as hepatitis types A through E, herpes, HIV, and Epstein-Barr
- Heavy metal toxicity (like mercury, for instance, from "silver" dental fillings or mercury amalgams)
- Undiagnosed food allergies; many people unknowingly suffer from lactose or gluten intolerance or may be allergic to corn or soy (common ingredients found in many processed foods), and undiagnosed food allergies have the potential to cause severe, chronic inflammation
- Environmental molds in the home or workplace; occult (hidden) mold can trigger the inflammation response in people who are susceptible to the toxins produced by various molds

Preventing Inflammation

Chronic inflammation often is seen in people who have diets with an unbalanced ratio of omega-6 and omega-3 essential fatty acids (EFAs). Increasing your intake of Omega-3 EFAs will help decrease the amount of internal inflammation. Foods rich in Omega-3 include fish, nuts such as walnuts, and seeds including chia and flaxseed. Although increasing your Omega-3 intake will improve your level of inflammation, it is also essential to eliminate inflammatory foods from the diet. Inflammatory foods are those that cause swelling and cellular dysregulation when consumed. Although all individuals do not react in the same manner to inflammatory foods, I continue to recommend an anti-inflammatory diet to my clients, especially in cases where autoimmune disease is present. By following an anti-inflammatory diet 80–90 percent of the time, the body is able to handle stress in a more efficient and effective manner. For those of you interested in eliminating inflammatory foods from your diet, they include but are not limited to these:

- Sugar
- Artificial sweeteners including aspartame (Equal or NutraSweet), sucralose (Splenda), saccharin (Sweet'N Low), Acesulfame K, dextrose, and others
- Table salt
- Processed and refined foods (anything in a can, box, or bag that is not in its original form from nature)
- Animal proteins including flesh, dairy products, animal fats and eggs
- Refined oils
- Fried foods
- Foods that contain gluten and/or gliadin, the protein present in rye, barley, triticale, spelt, wheat, farro, and einkorn
- Dairy products, including those from cow, buffalo, goat or sheep sources
- Unfermented soybean products such as soy flour, soy butter, soy cheese and other processed soy-based food items
- Alcoholic beverages
- Nightshade vegetables (the Solanaceae family of plants)—some of the major health complaints associated with nightshades include arthritis, irritable bowel syndrome (IBS), and fibromyalgia, which may occur because nightshade foods can remove calcium from bones and deposit it in soft tissue, causing inflammation; these plants also contain moderate amounts of nicotine, which can manipulate the bodies of those who by nature are sensitive - these foods to avoid include:
    - Tomato
    - Tomatillo
    - Eggplant

- White potato (excluding sweet potato)
- Peppers (includes hot and sweet varieties as well as spices like paprika, chili powder, cayenne, and Tabasco)
- Pimento
- Goji berry (wolfberry)
- Cape gooseberry/ground cherry
- Pepino
- Garden huckleberry

To fight inflammation, it is also important to resolve any nutrient deficiencies that may be present. This can be done by rebalancing and replenishing the intestinal flora with probiotics and taking trace minerals.

The more you can maximize the amount of fresh fruits and vegetables in your diet, the more balanced your body will be. Although I do not recommend a 100 percent raw food diet due to the malnutrition that may result with any restricted diet, it is important that you find a percentage of raw and fresh foods that is comfortable for you. It will be easier for you to incorporate more fresh foods if you have the right equipment and your pantry stocked with staples. It is also best to have a standard shopping list for easy reference. I have provided examples below.

BASIC KITCHEN EQUIPMENT

- Blender: High speed is best to create creamy dishes and blends, such as a Blendtec or Vitamix
- Stainless steel or glass bowls
- Bamboo cutting boards of various sizes
- Food processor (cup size varies): great for grating, slicing, and chopping; I like Cuisinart, Breville or KitchenAid
- Knives: professional-quality, stainless steel forged knives, such as Wusthof or Henckels, or comparable

Optional Kitchen Equipment

- Dehydrator: Excalibur 5 or 9 tray (these models have a built in timer, adjustable temperatures and provide enough surface area to create multiple recipes at a time).

- Juicer: I recommend the Angel Juicer because it allows me to keep my juice in the fridge for a few days without losing enzymes; however, the Hurom is another great juicer. For those just starting out, I recommend the Breville Compact, but, if using this juicer, be certain to consume your juice within a few hours to minimize nutrient loss.

- Salad spinner: OXO makes a great stainless steel spinner.

- Spiralizer: This is a fantastic kitchen tool that allows you to create spiral cuts and "noodles" out of vegetables and fruits such as zucchini, apples, carrots, etc. I prefer the Paderno brand because it has three or four blade options and works wonderfully.

WHEN PROBLEMS ARISE...

FOOD ALLERGIES AND INTOLERANCES

Writing a book has been a goal of mine for many years not only because I have had many requests, but, more importantly, because I wanted to write something that would help people feel better and restore their health. After much thought and consideration, I decided to start with this cookbook. As a naturopath, holistic nutritionist, and health counselor, my focus has always been working with those with special needs, including individuals battling *Candida albicans*, food allergies and sensitivities, cancers, arthritis, digestive diseases, diabetes, high cholesterol, hypertension, and fertility issues, as well as with those struggling with eating disorders. I work with hundreds of individuals though the course of a year, and I have come to realize there is an overwhelming need for education and guidance for not only living healthfully and naturally but also in preparing healthy, allergy-friendly, nurturing, and nutritious foods that are becoming less common in average households today.

When I was first diagnosed with multiple food sensitivities, I began experimenting with food and creating recipes free of gluten, dairy, eggs, peanuts, soy, and corn. Since then, I have changed my eating habits and am 100 percent free of gluten and dairy, and seldom eat soy or eggs, even if farm fresh. In rare instances, I consume organic, non-GMO corn. I generally avoid peanuts due to the fungal and aflatoxin poisons and eat mostly a vegan diet in the summer months. I occasionally will consume wild seafood and grass fed organic meats and poultry in the winter months.

Please realize that even if you are suffering from a health ailment, it does not mean you will never enjoy food again. I believe that individuality of each person, regardless of similarities to others, provides unique DNA, fingerprints, methylation capacities (the body's natural ability to detoxify), and lifestyles. This means no two individuals are alike, and, by acknowledging and accepting differentiation as an asset, we are able to embark on the redeeming journey to lasting health and wellness.

Food Allergy Elimination Trial

After eliminating suspecting food(s) from your diet for a period of no less than six months, you can try to reintroduce the offending food(s) to determine if the allergy is fixed or cyclical in nature.

I recommend keeping a complete and accurate food diary. Reintroduce the offending food on day 1 by eating a large amount at breakfast and a moderate amount at lunch. Avoid the offending food for four more days and monitor any symptoms.

Symptoms of food allergies can include the following:

- **Dermatological:** eczema, psoriasis, rashes, itching, acne
- **Gastrointestinal:** gas, bloating, abdominal pain, rectal bleeding, constipation, diarrhea, and other digestive diseases such as diverticulitis
- **General:** fatigue, mouth ulcers, headaches, low energy, nutritional deficiencies
- **Hormonal:** PMS symptoms, thyroid imbalance, insulin resistance, infertility, hot flashes
- **Immunological:** decreased ability to fight infections, delayed recovery time, autoimmune diseases
- **Learning challenges:** ADD/ADHD, behavioral problems, memory loss
- **Musculoskeletal:** muscle and joint pain, inflammation, trigger-point tenderness
- **Neurological:** brain fog, mood swings, anxiety, depression, sleep disturbance, anger issues
- **Respiratory:** chest tightness, runny nose, watering eyes, wheezing, chronic cough, sinusitis

If you do not experience symptoms, you may add the food back into your diet at a pace no more frequent than once every four days for at least six months unless symptoms reappear. After six months you can then add the food back in with more frequency if you remain symptom-free.

The top food intolerances that contribute to autoimmune disorders are gluten and dairy, and they will be covered here in detail.

Gluten

A gluten free diet is strongly recommended by medical professionals to treat celiac disease and wheat or gluten intolerance. You can readily find gluten free pasta, cereal, bread, waffles, pancakes, and cookies at most natural foods food stores, many supermarkets, and some local grocers. With online websites such as www.amazon.com, www.vitacost.com and www.drugstore.com, finding gluten free foods is quite simple. Gluten free foods include, but are not limited to, the following:

- Potatoes
- Buckwheat
- Oats (*must be labeled gluten free to avoid cross contamination)
- Corn/maize (please stick to non-GMO organic corn sources)
- Rice
- Wild rice
- Quinoa
- Amaranth
- Teff
- Millet
- Sorghum
- Tapioca or cassava
- Taro or yucca
- Arrowroot
- Beans
- Lentils
- Nuts and nut butters or flours
- Eggs (farm fresh, from grass fed chickens, are best)
- Fresh fruit
- Fresh vegetables
- Herbs and spices
- Meats and fish purchased without sauce or seasonings
- Homemade soups (avoid bouillon cubes, barley malt, and all types of pasta except those designated as gluten free)
- Juice (all-natural, 100 percent fruit juice)

Foods to Avoid

Wheat, kamut, couscous, farro, semolina, graham, spelt, einkorn, rye, and barley all contain gluten. Oats are generally avoided by those with gluten issues because often they are processed in mills and on equipment that also process grains containing gluten. Commonly used ingredients to avoid are flour, seitan, udon and soba noodles, imitation crab meat, bacon bits, food starch, dextrin, malto-dextrin, hydrolyzed or autolyzed yeast extract, vegetable protein, natural flavor, caramel color, gravy, brown rice syrup, barley enzymes (found in the majority of breakfast cereals), soy sauce, and distilled vinegar (malt vinegar). In general, the foods that are most likely to contain gluten, if not explicitly labeled as gluten free, are baked goods, malted beverages and beer, pasta, gravy or other sauces, meatballs, and meatloaf, as well as granola bars and other snack items.

Avoid Contamination

In addition, follow these tips to avoid contamination:

- Clean out cutlery drawers; they are great crumb collectors.
- Replace your old wooden spoons and cutting boards, as wood will absorb proteins from products containing gluten.
- Replace plastic storage containers since plastic is permeable and can absorb and release proteins and chemicals.
- Replace your nonstick pans and baking pans, cast iron pots and pans, and stoneware.
- Replace dish rags/sponges often.
- Replace your knife block and rolling pin if made of wood.
- Replace all electric appliances such as waffle makers that have a nonstick coating and grids where food can get stuck.
- Be sure to use a new toaster for gluten free foods only or buy toaster bags (do not use a toaster that's already been used to toast regular bread).
- Use squirt bottles for condiments like mayonnaise, mustard, jelly, etc. to avoid contamination from someone using a knife in the jar that was used on a gluten-containing food item. Also be wary of sugar canisters where double dipping could have contaminated your supply.

- At parties and events, avoid dips, salsas, and dipping oils to ensure you do not get cross contaminated from those who dip with gluten-based foods.
- Mark containers with "GF" on the lid of gluten free items so others know it is yours. There are stores online that offer washable GF stickers at a reasonable price.
- Clean food prep areas with Ava Anderson Non Toxic Hard Surface cleaner or use lemon juice, baking soda, and bleach if necessary.
- Wash your hands constantly, especially when living with those who do not follow a gluten free diet. Also be certain to wash common touchable items such as doorknobs, handles, and faucets to ensure no contamination occurs from daily exposure.

It is most important to make certain all skincare, body care, and household products are gluten free. The skin is our largest organ, and anything applied to the skin is absorbed into the blood in a matter of seconds. My favorite products are those made by Ava Anderson Non Toxic and can be found at www.nontoxicmomNY.com.

Grain free and Gluten free Baking Ingredients

Having food sensitivities does not mean you can never enjoy baked goods again. In fact, I have found that many of the allergy-friendly treats I create using the flours listed here have a better taste and texture and satiate me for longer periods of time. If you are willing to take a little bit of time to create your own baked goods, you can create any delicious treat that can be made with traditional flours. The trick is to try various flours to find the combination that best meets your personal needs and taste preferences. Unlike gluten-containing flours, you may need to combine three to five flours plus a gumming agent to create goods with good flavor and texture.

Whole Grain Flours

Amaranth flour: Amaranth flour is light in color, has a nutty flavor, and is high in protein, lysine, B vitamins, and moisture. It is a medium weight flour that is stickier than others and it browns quickly. Therefore, it should be used at lower temperatures for longer periods of time. It should be used in a mix with other flours, not alone, due to its earthy flavor.

Brown rice flour: This is the most commonly used gluten free flour. It has a faint nutty flavor and provides whole grain benefits to baked goods. It should be used in combination with other flours, otherwise a crumbly texture will result. It has a higher nutritional value than white rice flour. Superfine versions are best for baked goods.

Buckwheat flour: In the rhubarb family, buckwheat flour does not contain gluten despite its name. It has a deep flavor and a dark color and is high in calcium. It works well in breads, muffins, pancakes, crepes, and crackers, and contains all essential amino acids.

Chia seed meal: This is made from ground chia seeds. It adds omega-3 and calcium to baked goods. It provides a chewy texture and moistness to baked goods and adds extra protein and fiber. May be used as a replacement for eggs when mixed with warm water.

Coconut flour: Coconut flour offers structure to baked products and is extremely high in fiber and protein. It imparts a mild coconut flavor with sweetness ideal for desserts. It is highly absorbant so be certain to include ample liquid to recipe to prevent dryness. It can be grainy depending on the brand and should be used in combination with other flours.

Corn flour: Corn flour is also known as masa harina and is made from ground dried corn kernels. It offers a light texture and corn flavor and is available in many varieties, including yellow, purple, red, white, and blue.

Flaxseed meal: Made from ground flaxseeds, this adds omega-3, protein and fiber to baked goods. It can be used like chia seed flour and enables the baker to bake without using eggs, as it acts as a binding agent.

Garbanzo bean (chickpea) flour: This has a strong bean taste and is high in protein. It becomes rancid quickly and should be stored in the freezer. It should be used with other flours or alone in crepes and flatbreads. It can be used as a thickener or to provide denseness and structure to baked goods.

Gluten free oat flour: Oat flour adds texture and sweetness to baked goods. It offers fiber and B vitamins and allows you to use less sweetener in the recipe. It is wonderful in muffins, pancakes, and cookies. Make certain you buy gluten free oat flour to avoid cross contamination.

Mesquite flour: Mesquite flour is made from ground pods from the mesquite tree. It has a deep, rich flavor reminiscent of a combination of cinnamon, cocoa, and brown sugar with a hint of caramel and works wonderfully in baked goods that contain cocoa or coffee. It has a sweet taste and should be used with other flours as it is very dry and powdery.

Millet flour: Millet flour has a medium weight, and provides more structure than sorghum flour yet has a similarly sweet taste but with buttery notes. It is best in breads and savory goods in a mixture with other flours and is high in protein.

Nut flours (almond, cashew, etc.): Nut flours are made from nuts that are ground into a fine flour. They add texture and nuttiness to baked goods. High in protein and low in carbohydrates, these flours are exceptional for those with digestive issues and grain intolerance. Nut flours also can be used to bread meats or in lieu of bread crumbs in savory dishes like meatloaf. They should be stored in the freezer.

Potato flour: Potato flour should not be confused with potato starch. Potato flour is naturally heavy and provides elasticity and denseness. It is high in moisture and has a potato flavor.

Quinoa flour: Quinoa flour is a heavier flour that is high in protein and contains all essential amino acids. It has a slightly earthy taste and works best when combined with other flours. I don't use this flour often as I find the quinoa flavor overpowers most recipes.

Sorghum flour: Sorghum flour is a moderately light flour and has a very sweet flavor. It can result in crumbly goods and should be used in baked goods such as pie crusts, cookies, quick breads, and cakes. It contains high amounts of protein and fiber, with a wide array of B vitamins, and adds light texture to goods. I prefer light sorghum flour over dark sorghum flour.

Teff flour: Teff flour is high in protein, has a sweet honey-like flavor, and is available in ivory or dark varieties. It contains protein, iron, zinc, and calcium. It adds body to baked goods and can be used as thickner due to its sticky nature.

White rice flour: White rice flour is starchy with a mild, sweet taste. It can be used as a starch and adds sponginess to baked goods but has little nutrient value. Used alone in baked goods, it causes a dry and crumbly product.

Starches

Arrowroot: Arrowroot is a thickener that can be used in place of tapioca, potato, or cornstarches. It softens and lightens baked goods but can get gummy if used in excess. It is more expensive than some of the other starchy flours.

Cornstarch: Cornstarch is a thickener with little flavor. It makes baked goods crispy and lightens up flour blends. It is good for thickening sauces or to make crumbly baked goods such as shortbread.

Potato starch: Potato starch imposes little to no flavor as long as paired with other flours and should not be confused with potato flour. It is used to thicken, primarily in soups and stews, as well as provide lightness, lift and crispiness to baked goods.

Sweet rice flour: This is also known as mochi. It is ground from brown or white sticky rice and so is more often used in baked goods, as it becomes thick and extremely gummy if boiled. It is mild and tasteless and provides crispness without grit. It can also be used to dredge meats and fish before pan searing. It is wonderful for making gravies as it does not clump or impart flavor. It works very well in combination with coconut and nut flours.

Tapioca starch: Tapioca starch is the same as tapioca flour. It is a starch that is used to thicken without added flavor and lends crispness to baked goods. Too much can cause a gluey and gummy product so it is best combined with other starchy flours if a light, airy texture is desired.

Binders and Gelling Agents

Gelatin: Gelatin is a readily available alternative to guar and xanthan gums. It provides structure and density to gluten free products. It helps provide sponginess to gluten free baked goods and helps retain moisture in the product when used as a binder. It can help provide fluffiness to cakes. I don't use gelatin very often because items tend to become rubbery unless a gelatinous texture is desired.

Guar Gum: Guar Gum is a bean-based product that emulsifies and thickens substances. It provides softness and elasticity to baked goods. In my experience, it works best in cold foods like dressings, ice creams and puddings. It has less elasticity than xanthan gum so more guar gum may be needed in some recipes. It is much more affordable than xanthan gum as well.

Xanthan Gum: Xanthan Gum is a polysaccharide created through bacterial fermentation derived from corn that is often used to thicken or gel substances. It is frequently used in gluten free baking to replicate the stretchy and elastic qualities present in gluten. It seems to work the best in gluten free baked goods and is essential in any gluten free yeast bread.

Dairy (Casein/Whey)

I have concluded from my research and through personal experiences with myself and clients that dairy is not a healthy part of a lifestyle designed for optimal wellness. It is interesting to note that humans are the only mammal who do not wean completely off milk. Instead, once we have weaned from our mother's milk, we switch to cow's milk, which is designed for a five-hundred-pound calf. In short, human breast milk is for humans, cow's milk is for cows. Contrary to what the commercials on television tell us, our body cannot fully utilize the calcium or protein found in cow's milk, even in fermented forms such as yogurt and kefir, often touted to be wonderful sources of calcium. In addition, dairy products are extremely mucous forming and are one of the most inflammatory foods available to us today. It is worth mentioning that many studies have found that casein, a protein found in dairy products, contributes to breast cancer (Vieira FG1, 2011). I cannot make the choice for you, but if you do intend to consume dairy, I recommend consuming grass fed, raw, and organic cow, goat, or sheep milk so that the enzymes helpful in breaking down the protein and sugar in the milk are still intact and viable. I find that goat and sheep milks are more similar in macro- and micronutrients to human breast milk than cow's milk, making it easier for the human body to absorb the nutrients. Goat and sheep milks are also lower in casein, a milk protein that often causes allergic reaction in those sensitive to cow's milk. No more than sixteen ounces of milk for children aged three or less or twenty-four ounces for those older than four should be consumed, as the phosphorus in the milk can deplete iron stores, leading to chronic health issues including anemia (Physicians Committee for Responsible Medicine, n.d.), potential bone loss, and blood disorders.

Calcium is readily available in many foods besides dairy products (Academy of Nutrition and Dietetics, 2014), and it is 100 percent absorbable by the human body when plant based. Some incredible and delicious sources of calcium include these:

- Hempseed milk (1 cup contains 460 mg)
- Blackstrap molasses (2 tablespoons contains 400 mg)
- Collard greens (1 cup contains over 350 mg)
- Fortified orange juice (1 cup contains 300 mg)
- Amaranth (1 cup contains 275 mg)
- Turnip greens (1 cup contains 250 mg)
- Tempeh (1 cup contains 215 mg)
- Fortified nondairy milk (1 cup contains 200–300 mg)
- Kale (1 cup contains 180 mg)
- Edamame (1 cup contains 175 mg)
- Tahini (2 tablespoons contains 130 mg)
- Navy beans (1 cup contains 125 mg)
- Great northern beans (1 cup contains 120 mg)
- Figs (½ cup contains 120 mg)
- Raw fennel (1 medium bulb contains 115 mg)
- Broccoli (1 cup contains 95 mg)
- Almond butter (2 tablespoons contains 85 mg)
- Adzuki beans (1 cup contains 65 mg)
- Black currants (1 cup contains 62 mg)

- Artichokes (1 medium artichoke contains 55 mg)
- Oranges (1 orange contains between 50 and 60 mg)
- Blackberries (1 cup contains 40 mg)
- Dried apricots (½ cup contains 35 mg)
- Dates (½ cup contains 35 mg)
- Roasted sesame seeds (1 oz. contains 35 mg)

Milk Alternatives

Coconut Milk

Coconut milk is my favorite nondairy milk because it looks like dairy milk. In addition, it can be creamy, especially when homemade, which is highly recommended. It withstands hot temperatures and is one of the least allergenic milk alternatives on the market today. It is low calorie and is high in caprylic and lauric acids, which are natural antimicrobial agents. Coconut milk is made by removing the meat of the coconut and blending it with the liquids contained within the coconut or purified water. It does have a moderate saturated fat content, but because it is plant based, it does not contribute to poor health. Coconut milk is rich in iron and can assist with maintaining blood sugar levels. The downside is that coconut milk is not very high in protein.

If you choose to purchase coconut milk, you can buy it in a can or aseptic container. I prefer the canned milk when looking for a rich, creamy alternative for soups, desserts, and creamy spreads. In addition, the cream sitting atop the milk can be whipped into a delightful heavy cream alternative. Ultimately, making your own coconut milk is best so you avoid additives, including gums and carrageenan, but if you want to go halfway, many markets sell powdered coconut cream that you can blend with water to create a delicious, creamy milk that is free from preservatives and emulsifiers.

Almond Milk

Another favorite milk alternative is almond milk, which is made by blending whole almonds or almond meal with water and then straining the pulp (which makes a great flour). Almond milk is rich in calcium, protein, zinc, and iron and is free of saturated fat. It is also low calorie. Be very selective if buying almond milks in the store, however, because many contain other fillers, preservatives, and emulsifiers, as well as high amounts of sodium. Besides, fresh almond milk is much creamier and so much more delicious. Almond milk works well for baking and is wonderful warmed and sweetened with raw honey on a chilly night.

Cashew Milk

Cashew milk is another favorite due to its creamy nature. It is now available in stores; however, it does contain additives. A wonderful aspect of making your own cashew milk is that it can be made in seconds. Cashews do not require soaking (although I often soak them to release the enzymes) and can be blended with water—no straining required. It is thick, creamy, and neutral in taste, especially when compared to some of the other milk alternatives. Cashew milk is rich in B vitamins, potassium, and zinc and extremely rich in magnesium, a mineral in which many people are deficient. Cashews are also low in calories and fat when compared to other nuts and seeds ounce for ounce, so rotating cashew milk into your milk alternative repertoire is highly recommended.

Sunflower Seed Milk

Sunflower milk is fairly new in the markets today and is made from soaked sunflower seeds that are blended with water. It is pale gray in color and is fairly thin in consistency, so it is not recommended in certain applications where thickening is necessary. Sunflower milk is a good choice for those who have developed sensitivities to tree nuts because sunflower seeds are not as allergenic and offer folic acid and vitamins B5 and B6 to increase energy. Sunflower seeds are known for fighting inflammation and can help with joint mobility and building strong bones. Sunflower seeds contain arginine, which helps with blood flow and can improve heart health. They are also rich in vitamin E and can help with skin issues including eczema and acne.

Again, I recommend making your own sunflower seed milk from sprouted sunflower seeds so you can maximize the nutrients and enzymes present in the milk. I frequently blend in dates for sweetness and alcohol-free vanilla extract or vanilla bean for a more balanced pleasant taste.

Flax Milk

Flaxseed milk is available in many major grocery stores, but it is easy to make at home from soaked raw flaxseeds. Flaxseed milk is extremely low in calories and is one of the best sources of omega-3 fatty acids (about 1,200 mg), calcium, and alpha linolenic acids (ALA). It also contains iron, making it a good choice for vegans or vegetarians who may suffer from anemia. Flax milk has a very neutral taste, and I think it tastes very similar to skim milk. It is thin in consistency and has a slightly opaque white color. Flaxseeds have anticancer properties, are a natural estrogen that can balance hormones, and encourage brain and heart health.

Hempseed Milk

Hempseed milk is perhaps my favorite seed-based milk alternative because of the high nutrient content. It is rich in omega-3s, contains ten essential amino acids, and is higher in protein (24 percent) than the alternatives. Although it is not a popular milk from a taste aspect for many, it is my favorite milk from a nutrition standpoint. Hempseeds also contain omega-6 fats, which enhance the health of our skin, hair, and fingernails. Hempseed is a complete protein, is hypoallergenic, and is easy to digest and assimilate, making it ideal in a pre-workout smoothie. It is even thought that hempseeds offer natural sunscreen protection.

It does taste good particularly when homemade because it is nutty and earthy in flavor, making it delicious in puddings and ice cream. I prefer to make my own simply because many of the hempseed milks on the market today are very high in sugars, and if you make it at home, you can use more natural sweeteners. I generally do not strain my hemp milk when I make it because hempseeds are a wonderful source of fiber and iron and I prefer to keep as many nutrients as I can in the milk. If you have a good blender hempseed milk tends to blend smoothly and without fuss.

Quinoa Milk

Quinoa milk is not as well known, but it is now on grocery store shelves. It is remarkably similar to rice milk in taste and texture but has a darker color. Quinoa is a complete protein with plenty of amino acids and is rich in vitamins D and E. It is very creamy but has an earthy flavor that enhances coffee and other beverages and is delicious in breakfast porridge. I like to make my own quinoa milk so that I can add in other flavors such as vanilla or almond extract or more simply blend in other ingredients such as pecans. It does require straining, however, to keep a smooth consistency.

Oat Milk

Oat milk is made by soaking oats and then blending the oats with fresh water in a blender. Oat milk offers a high-protein, low-fat alternative to dairy milk. Oats are rich in phytochemicals that may protect the body against cancer, heart disease, and skin conditions. If purchasing oat milk in an aseptic container, make sure it is gluten free, as many brands include barley malt as a sweetener or do not use certified gluten free oats. Oat milk does have an oatmeal taste, so it may not be suitable for all culinary uses.

Oats can help with sugar and nicotine cravings by regulating the body's stress response system. Oats, particularly steel-cut oats, help nourish those with depression and may help lower cholesterol. They contain rich phytochemicals that slow the aging process and aid digestion, making oat milk a good choice for those with sensitive digestive tracts.

Hazelnut Milk

Hazelnut milk is another tree nut–based milk that you can find in specialty health stores. It has a strong hazelnut taste and is ivory in color. I find that hazelnut milk can be overpowering, especially when used in baking, so if I make this milk at home, I prefer to combine it with other ingredients such as cashew or coconut to balance the flavor. Hazelnuts are wonderful for heart health and for lowering cholesterol. They contain all the B vitamins and are especially rich in folate, vitamin E, fiber, calcium, and zinc, an essential nutrient for strong immunity and reproductive health. In addition, hazelnuts are very nourishing; I often use hazelnut oil on my skin, as it absorbs nicely, is not greasy, and smells nice.

Be certain to check the packaging if purchasing at a store, as some hazelnut milks do contain barley malt, which is not gluten free.

Rice Milk

Rice milk is made from simmered brown rice and water that is pureed in a blender and then strained. It is highly available in most areas across the country. Rice milk is not as nutritious as other nondairy milks, but still is cholesterol free, contains B vitamins, and offers protein. I generally use caution in using rice milk because not only is it a thinner milk alternative that does not thicken well without adding other thickening agents, but it has been found to contain moderate amounts of inorganic and organic arsenic, even when organic (Reporter, 2014).

Rice milk is high in calories and natural starch, however is sweet in flavor naturally, making it a better alternative to those who are transitioning to nondairy milks. It is also the most hypoallergenic among all the milk alternatives and is the lowest in fat as well.

Soy Milk

Soy milk is made from dried soybean flour and water. From a nutrition standpoint, soy milk has an impressive nutritional label when it comes to protein and calcium and is rich in potassium, which can help one avoid stroke or high blood pressure. However, I generally avoid soy due to the phytoestrogen properties of soy, which may be harmful to women, men, and children alike. In addition, soy products including soy milk can be difficult to digest, causing gas and bloating. It is important to note too that unless soy milk is certified organic, it is likely to be genetically modified and, therefore, an unnatural food source. Soy is also one of the top ten allergens in America today.

Other Alternative Milks

You can generally make a milk alternative from anything, including potatoes or bananas; however, it may not be tasty or serve a wide variety of purposes. For instance, I have made banana milk by blending a banana and eight to twelve ounces of water together in a blender until smooth to top cereal when staying at a friend's home where only dairy milk was available. You could even try potato milk, made from mashed potatoes and water. It has a very neutral flavor, blends nicely, and is a great addition to creamy soups and in baking. I generally make my milk out of nuts, seeds, grain, or coconut as I have found that they have a richer flavor, have higher nutritional values, are more versatile, and are readily available if I need to pick up the ingredients at the store.

Additional Modifications

Egg Alternatives

Flax or Chia Egg

A flax or chia egg is made by simply combining three tablespoons of warm water with one tablespoon of ground seed and allowing to sit for a few minutes before utilizing in a recipe. This combination acts as a binder and works well in baked goods and breads. Using flax or chia eggs can cause a dryer product so adding a few extra tablespoons of liquid may be necessary for the desired texture.

Psyllium Husk

Found in the fiber section at your health food store, psyllium is an extremely absorbant ingredient that works well as a binder when you want height in your product without changing the texture of the product itself. It adds a good amount of fiber and can add crunch to homemade crackers. It is a great substitute for those recipes where chia or flax eggs cause gumminess.

Nut or Seed Butters

Nut butters work well in heavier baked goods with short cooking times such as brownies, granola, whole grain crackers or granola and protein bars. They bind well, add fat, moisture and richness to products with a delicate nutty flavor.

Egg Replacer Powder

There are a number of egg replacer powders on the market today. If you are avoiding dairy be certain to avoid those that contain milk powder. In general, these powders are a combination of starches and act as a leavener in cookies, breads and pancakes.

Mashed Fruits

Mashed fruits act well as a binder or when added moisture is desired in a recipe. Some examples of mashed fruits include banana, applesauce, or avocado. These work best in sweet baked goods, cakes and muffins because they are light and neutral in flavor (except for bananas). I suggest removing 1/8 to 1/4 of the wet ingredients in the recipe to make up for the moisture in the mashed fruit. You can also use pureed soaked fruits such as dates, apricots and figs in recipes that can benefit from extra sweetness and crunch. Because dried fruits tend to caramelize when baking, they can offer some extra crunch and flavor in cookies, brownies and other desserts where crispy edges may be desired.

Mashed Sweet Potato or Squash

Mashed sweet potato, regular potato, squash or pumpkin puree work the same as the mashed fruits. These work best in sweet baked goods and quick breads that have a denser texture. Again, I suggest removing 1/8 to 1/4 of your wet ingredients in the recipe to make up for the moisture in the mashed vegetable.

Baking Powder

Baking powder performs as a leavener and works best in pancakes, cookies and breads. It does add quite a bit of sodium to the recipe unless you are using the Hain brand which is potassium based instead of sodium based.

Tapioca flour or arrowroot

Tapioca flour and arrowroot are flours made from whole foods that offer an exceptional amount of starch to a recipe. These act as thickeners and can be used in puddings, gravies or other thick sauces. They are also used in baking to help lighten a recipe or offer a pleasant texture without adding flavor.

Silken Tofu or Tofu Puree, or Non-Dairy Yogurt

These wet substances behave as either a binder or thickener or provide additional moisture when desired in a recipe. I most often use these in creamy pie bases, or in muffins, cakes and breads that need extra moisture.

Unflavored Gelatin

Unflavored gelatin is a great substance to use in baking when a binder or firming agent is needed. It is also wonderful for making creamy pies and helps making slicing possible. It can also be used in making homemade jellies and jams.

Sugar Replacements

Dates and other dried fruits, in whole or dried and ground form: Naturally sweet fruits can be used in raw or dehydrated forms. Fruit sugars are made from dried fruits that are either ground or soaked. Pastes are created when fruits are pureed with water to form a thick, creamy paste that can be used interchangeably with sugar or other liquid sweeteners. Some fruits that make exceptionable sweeteners include dates, bananas, prunes, or raisins. I often use date puree to sweeten oatmeal or to replace liquid sweeteners such as honey or maple syrup in baking for a more dynamic flavor.

Maple products: Maple syrup is boiled-down sap from maple trees. It has an extremely sweet and pleasant flavor. The darker the syrup, the better the nutrition, so I recommend Grade B 100 percent organic maple syrup (sometimes called Grade A Very Dark) from New York, Vermont or Canada. Maple syrup is high in calcium and manganese and is available in granular form, which imparts a lovely maple flavoring to baked goods.

Honey and bee products: These are products that are made from bees and flower nectars and come in a variety of flavors and varieties. Honey contains enzymes, nutrients, and B vitamins that build immune health. It can be used topically on burns and wounds to hasten healing, encourages bowel health, and is a wonderful remedy for seasonal allergies and for coughs and colds, especially those deep in the lungs. Be sure to use local honey in the raw form.

Stevia**: Stevia is an herb native to South America that resembles basil. It is up to three hundred times sweeter than sugar. Best used in the natural green form, as the white versions are processed, it is also available as a liquid or in tablet form. Stevia can be bitter, so try various brands before giving up on it, as it is the best sweetener, in my opinion, in terms of health. Make certain to purchase 100 percent whole stevia leaf extract that contains no other additives or fillers such as dextrin, erythritol, sugar, or maltodextrin.

Lo han**: Made from monk fruit, lo han is found in liquid or powdered form. It is up to three hundred times sweeter than sugar with little aftertaste. It does not raise blood sugar and helps balance the bitter aftertaste when used in conjunction with stevia. Again, be certain to find pure lo han, not one containing other ingredients.

Xylitol**: Xylitol is also known as birch sugar when 100 percent birch is used. Many xylitol products on the market also contain corn that may be genetically modified, so seek out 100 percent birch xylitol. It contains approximately one-third fewer calories than sugar. Because it is a sugar alcohol, it can cause gas and bloating. Xylitol is known to prevent tooth decay and is used in many toothpastes, mouthwashes, and chewing gum because of its dental health benefits. I recommend using this product in strict moderation, as it is still processed.

Erythitol**: This is a sugar alcohol made from fermented corn or sugar. It has little health benefit, although it is free of calories. It can cause gas, bloating, and digestive ailments. I recommend using this ingredient in strict moderation because of the processing required to transform it into usable form.

Yacon syrup**: This product originated in Peru and is a thick, rich syrup made from the yacon root. It is a low glycemic sweetener that is an FOS (fructooligosaccharide)—an indigestible starch. It acts as a prebiotic regulating digestive health. It is low in calories and is an ample source of potassium.

Vegetable glycerin**: This is an extremely sweet thick syrup derived from coconut and palm oils. It should be used vary sparingly due to its extreme bitterness.

Coconut palm sugar or nectar: This is made from coconut sap. It is rich in potassium and magnesium and low on the glycemic index. Processed at low temperatures to retain nutrient benefits and neutral in pH, it is available in syrup or granular form. It is mild in flavor and tastes similar to brown sugar.

Sucanat, turbinado, and other less refined sugars: These are less processed sugars that are not bleached and have larger granules. They are still sugar, which is best avoided as it can lead to chronic inflammation in the body.

Brown rice syrup: This syrup is made from brown rice that is ground and cooked over high heat to produce a syrup with a mild flavor, reminiscent of caramel. Be certain to buy gluten free versions only as others contain barley malt. I also use caution when using this ingredient as it tends to contain higher levels of arsenic due to the natural processing of rice.

Molasses: Molasses is a highly nutritious syrup derived from reduced sugar that is rich in iron, zinc, calcium, and magnesium. It has a very strong flavor that is more concentrated the darker the syrup. It helps facilitate fat and cellular metabolism and provides the cells with energy. Blackstrap molasses is a wonderful food to battle anemia due to its rich iron content, and manganese makes it a highly effective antioxidant for battling free radicals. It is also known to boost energy, improve digestion, and aid in weight loss.

Fruit juice concentrate**:** Concentrated fruit juices form a thick syrup that is all natural. It is intensely sweet so a little goes a long way. It can be made from juice of any fruit. Wax Orchards makes a fruit juice concentrate in a jar.

Agave nectar: This comes from the agave cactus, is high in fructose, is processed at low temperatures, has a neutral flavor, and is 35 to 40 percent sweeter than sugar. When using agave in baked goods, lower the baking temperature fifteen to twenty-five degrees for best results. It is processed in the same fashion as high fructose corn syrup, which involves the use of potent filtration chemicals and has been linked to miscarriage (Nagel, 2009). I generally avoid agave nectar for this reason.

Inulin powder**: This is another FOS powder, in this case made from chicory root. It has similar benefits to yacon root. It promotes healthy bowel function and reduces gastrointestinal inflammation.

** Candida friendly

Nuts/Seeds

Raw nuts and seeds are wonderful snack foods that contain a wide range of essential vitamins and minerals. They are a food source of healthy, unsaturated fats and can help with appetite regulation, as well as weight maintenance. Nuts contain fiber and high amounts of protein per ounce to encourage fat burning in the body. Nuts and seeds are best consumed raw, as the roasted process can cause the delicate oils to become rancid and harmful. Unless you have an allergy to nuts, I recommend consuming a maximum of one-quarter cup of loose nuts or seeds or two tablespoons of raw nut or seed butter each day due to their high fat and vitamin E content. These nutrient powerhouses are a great snack for those with low blood sugar or diabetes, as they contain little, if any, natural sugar. Nut meals and flours can be used successfully in gluten free or grain free baking with wonderful and delicious results. In addition, nut butters can be used as a fat replacement, to thicken sauces or dressings, and as flavor enhancers. Nuts also add healthy fiber, essential fats and nutrients, and protein to any dish. If nut allergies are a concern, seed flours and seed butters can be used in equal exchange for their nut counterparts.

It is important to note that each nut has a very different nutrient structure; therefore, rotating the types of nuts and seeds you consume ensures proper vitamin and mineral balance.

To soak or not to soak...

Although eating a moderate amount of nuts and seeds daily is healthy, soaking them in raw form stimulates the process of germination, which increases the vitamin C, vitamin B, and beta carotene content. Soaking may also neutralize phytic acid, a substance that can inhibit absorption of calcium, magnesium, iron, copper, and zinc. Nuts also contain enzymes that can hamper proper digestion and assimilation, which can be neutralized by soaking. Generally the best nuts and seeds for soaking include almonds (about eight hours), cashews and sunflower seeds (two hours), and walnuts and pecans (about one hour). If you choose to soak your nuts and seeds, please be certain to rinse the nuts/seeds until the water runs clear to remove any residue.

If the idea of soaking your nuts and seeds seems too time consuming or overwhelming, simply rinsing nuts before eating can help remove much of the processing debris.

Name of Nut/Seed	Key Nutrients	Acid/Alkaline
Almonds	Vitamin E, Calcium, Magnesium, Potassium	Alkaline
Walnuts	Omega-3 fatty acids, Glutathione	High Acid
Pecans	Vitamins A, and E, Zinc, Phosphorus, Folate	Moderate Acid
Cashews	Magnesium, Phosphorus, Iron, B vitamins	Moderate Acid
Chestnuts	Manganese, Copper	Alkaline
Hazelnuts	Vitamins E, B1, B2, B3 and B6	Alkaline
Pistachios	Phosphorus	High Acid
Brazil nuts	Selenium, Phosphorus, Choline	Alkaline
Macadamia nuts	Essential fatty acids	Alkaline
Coconut	Manganese, Copper	Neutral
Flaxseed	ALA, Lingans, Iron	Alkaline
Hemp seeds	Omega-3 and Omega-6 fatty acids	Alkaline
Chia seeds	Calcium, Omega-3 fatty acids	Alkaline
Pine nuts	Zinc, Vitamins B1 and B3	Low Acid
Sunflower seeds	Folic acid, Vitamins B5 and B6	Low Acid
Pumpkin seeds	Vitamin A, Zinc, Iron	Low Acid
Apricot kernels	Vitamin E	Alkaline
Sesame seeds	Calcium, Iron, Phytic acid, B Vitamins, Niacin	Low Acid
Poppy seeds	Zinc	Low Acid

WHEN AWAY FROM HOME...

DEFENSIVE EATING AND DINING OUT

Eating out can be a nightmare for those with food allergies, but if you prepare yourself there is no reason why you cannot feel free to dine out safely. I recommend that you plan ahead of time by contacting the restaurant in advance to speak with management or the head chef or finding their menu online to review your menu choices before arriving at the restaurant. By being prepared, you are able to ask how the meals are prepared (i.e., in a separate area, with special cooking utensils, in a designated kitchen, etc.). Many restaurants today are aware of the increasing number of individuals with allergies and sensitivities and want to please you. They believe if you have a pleasant dining experience with them, you will tell others with similar concerns, and they will have an advantage over other restaurants that do not offer accommodations. Public awareness efforts have led to victories such as celiac disease being recognized by the Americans with Disability Act (ADA), which requires restaurants to make a reasonable accommodation to those requesting modification.

For gluten and dairy free dining, it is best to avoid fast-food restaurants not only because their meal options are made of low-quality ingredients, but because they use so many fillers and preservatives that it is nearly impossible to ensure a product is gluten and/or dairy free. They also prepare your food in the same work area as the allergenic foods, increasing the risk of exposure. Some of the larger, midscale chains, such as Chipotle, do offer options and menus that can be viewed online. They also have vowed to serve fresh foods that are GMO and antibiotic free, which lessens the chances that hidden allergens are contained. However, it is important to note that restaurants such as these have a higher potential for cross contamination as they are working quickly to prepare a meal for a line of people. When I get to the front of the line, I politely explain that I have allergies and ask them to change their gloves, and as I order, I look at what I am selecting so I can avoid cross contamination. For example, if I order a salad, I oversee their ingredients to see if there are visible contaminants. For example, if the guacamole has sour cream or cheese that has dripped into the container, I will avoid the guacamole or ask for fresh guacamole from a new container. Scraping off the contaminating food does not ensure it is safe.

When visiting finer dining establishments, there are a few key things to remember. The first is never to order a dish that says it has gravy, au jus, sauce, or other garnishes. Order your protein simply grilled, baked, or broiled, being certain to ask your server to make sure it is not cooked in butter or dredged in flour. This is when it is most appropriate to call in advance so you can talk to a manager, rather than relying on wait staff to ensure your health!

The second tip is to order lots of vegetables and request that they be served raw or steamed. You can also ask for them to be sautéed or grilled in extra virgin olive oil, but make sure to ask, again, that no butter, butter-flavored cooking sprays, or margarine (which contains milk proteins) be used. Many restaurants will offer to cook your protein and/or veggies on a sheet of aluminum foil to ensure you are not cross contaminated from the grill itself.

When ordering salads, always be certain to specify that you are gluten and dairy free, even if the salad does not list those ingredients, as restaurants do not always list every ingredient, including those such as croutons or shaved cheese. Feel free to offer examples by indicating that you are dairy and gluten free and would like ABC Salad, with no cheese, croutons, or candied nuts (which will likely be roasted in butter or cream). Be wary of salad dressings, and order simple oil and vinegar or ask for some limes or lemons to squeeze over your salad. If you frequent the restaurant, you may be able to inquire about vinaigrettes that would meet your dietary needs. In worse-case scenarios, top your salad with salsa, watered-down hummus, or mashed-up avocado or dairy free guacamole, if available.

Obviously do not order any menu options that contain gluten or dairy, such as pastas, fried foods, or cheese-filled pastries. Dessert options are limited when dining out, and it is extremely important not to be fooled by the gluten free flourless cake, as it is mostly made with eggs and butter (which is made from cow's milk and is therefore a dairy product). Rather, ask if they have fresh fruit or sorbet to sweeten your palate after a meal. I often keep a vegan chocolate bar in my purse for when sweet cravings kick in after a meal and there are no safe dessert options in which to indulge.

Traveling with Food Allergies/Intolerances

Always be ready by packing your own snacks and meals when traveling, especially by airplane. Airlines may offer some type of gluten free snack, but it is less likely to be dairy, egg, or soy free as well. By being prepared with a few provisions in your carry-on bag, you can avoid illness due to cross contamination. Please remember that most airlines will not allow you to travel with liquids, gels, or pastes over four ounces. This includes oatmeal, applesauce, nut or peanut butter, hummus, guacamole, smoothies, and so forth.

The best foods to bring are those that will offer nutrition and satiate your appetite until you get to your destination, where you can find more variety. Having snacks and meals that are higher in nutrition will allow you to have more energy, be more relaxed, and enjoy your trip. It will also keep your body balanced during the stressful travel event.

The following is a list of allergy-friendly meals you can prepare for your trip:

- Brown rice or organic corn tortilla stuffed with veggies, grilled chicken, tuna or Sunflower Veggie Spread (see Snacks)
- Brown rice sushi with gluten free soy sauce packets (San-J)
- Large green salad with Sweet Turkey Meatballs, Salmon Loaf or Beanloaf chunks (see Entrees)
- Simple Veggie Burger (see Entrees) on gluten free hamburger bun
- Creamy Cinnamon Bean Dip (see Snacks) on rice cakes
- Sarah's Protein Pancake (see Breakfast)
- Cauliflower Salad (see Sides) with grilled fish or chicken

Remember to include sides such as chopped raw veggies, fresh fruits, trail mix, rice cakes, and a few pieces of dark (eighty percent or more) chocolate.

Keep these snack ideas in mind:

- Cheesy Kale Chips (see Snacks)
- Baby food packets (under four ounces)
- Chickpea Poppers (see Snacks)
- Whole fruit like apples, grapes, berries, oranges, etc.
- Grain Free Crackers with Roasted Red Pepper Hummus (see Snacks)

- Any of the muffin recipes (see Breakfast)
- Vitality Balls or Protein Bars (see Snacks)
- Homemade trail mix with nuts, seeds, vegan chocolate chips, goji berries, etc.

What If I Get Contaminated?

Detoxifying and Cleansing Safely

We live in a toxic world through the air we breathe, the foods we eat, and the chemicals we absorb from our environment and home. Our organs are capable of naturally methylating the toxins out of our body on a daily basis; however, our toxic burden has become much greater over the past several decades, and sometimes our body needs assistance in carrying out the process of eliminating harmful substances from the body. If the body does not have ample nutrients, it cannot detoxify efficiently or effectively, and, as a result, toxins recirculate through the body and then are stored. Eventually, the body becomes damaged and presents with diagnosed medical conditions.

Examples of toxicity include these:

- Digestive complications including indigestion, constipation, diarrhea, gas, bloating
- Neurological issues including migraines or headaches, foggy thinking, disorientation
- Weight gain
- Metallic taste in mouth
- Joint and muscle soreness, stiffness, and aches
- Acne
- Fatigue and lethargy
- Ringing in the ears
- Excess mucus and drainage
- Skin rashes and hives, eczema
- Bad breath and body odor
- Circles under the eyes

Our main detoxification organ is the liver, and all substances ingested are processed through the liver. Nutrients essential for proper liver function include these:

- Glutathione
- Sulfur
- Vitamin C
- Vitamin B6
- Zinc
- Antioxidants including turmeric and resveratrol
- Fiber
- Pure water

Ways to Detoxify

- Limit chemical exposure and use non toxic personal care and cleaning products.
- Purify your air and water.
- Eat a well-balanced diet.
- Do a seasonal cleanse program (up to four times per year) under the supervision of a professional.
- Drink cleansing herb tea like dandelion, milk thistle, burdock, or nettles.
- Clean up your emotional health.
- Drink distilled water with a light diet for four days. Fresh organic lemon slices will also assist the liver in dumping toxins.

RECIPES

BREAKFAST

Perfect Gluten free Zucchini Bread

Makes 4 small loaves

I love quick breads because not only are they speedy, but they can be a healthier way to enjoy a sweet treat. I also love that they can be used for breakfast, snacks or an after-dinner treat. I make all quick breads using this blend of flours because of the sweetness and smooth texture.

Dry Ingredients:

1 cup Sarah's All Purpose Flour Blend

¼ cup coconut flour

¼ cup almond flour

2 Tbsp gluten free oat flour

1 Tbsp baking powder

2 tsp cinnamon

½ tsp xanthan gum

½ tsp baking soda

½ tsp sea salt

¼ tsp ground nutmeg

Wet Ingredients:

1 ½ small zucchini

¼ cup coconut oil

¼ cup applesauce or other fruit puree

½ cup organic brown sugar

¼ cup coconut palm sugar

Egg replacer for 2 eggs

2 packets stevia

1 tsp apple cider vinegar

¼ cup coconut milk (or another unsweetened dairy or non-dairy milk)

Preheat oven to 350° F. Grease four mini-loaf pans.

In a large bowl, whisk all of the dry ingredients together well. In a blender, combine the wet ingredients together and run until smooth. Pour the wet ingredients into the dry and mix together well using a whisk or wooden spoon until the batter thickens.

Evenly distribute batter amongst the four loaf pans. Smooth the tops with your finger if desired (I always do this). Bake for 40 to 45 minutes. Place onto a wire rack to cool. Remove from pan after about 10 minutes and cool completely before serving.

Crockpot Steel Cut Oats

Serves 8

If you are short on time in the morning, whether it be you like to sleep in, or you have kids to get off to school, this recipe saves you time and has a pleasant aroma that lofts throught the house upon rising in the morning. Feel free to experiment with various types of dried fruit, nuts and spices for a change in essence.

2 cups gluten free steel cut oats

6 cups water

4 cups organic apple juice

½ tsp sea salt

2 Tbsp coconut oil (optional)

½ cup dried fruit (raisins, prunes, apricots, dates)

1 Tbsp vanilla or gluten free maple extract

Maple syrup or organic brown sugar to taste

Place all ingredients in a 6 quart slow cooker and stir. Cover and cook on low for 7 hours. Note: If using smaller slow cooker, it is best to halve the recipe to ensure proper cooking.

Simple Pancake Mix

Makes 8 - 4" pancakes

Pancakes are the most popular recipe that I have requested. I totally understand as I grew up eating pancakes on the weekends, but they were a special treat. Pancakes are great simply because you make them in any flavor you wish, but I try to stick with a simple version like this, and add flavorings on top. The leftover pancakes freeze well and can be used to make breakfast sandwiches.

¼ cup brown rice flour

¼ cup gluten free oat flour

¼ cup coconut flour

¼ cup potato starch

1 Tbsp coconut palm sugar

1 Tbsp ground chia seed

2 tsp baking powder

½ tsp baking soda

½ tsp sea salt

Combine all ingredients in a large bowl and whisk to combine. Store in a glass jar in the pantry.

Preparation instructions:

Using a whisk, add the following ingredients to 1 cup of pancake mix. Allow batter to sit 2 to 3 minutes before cooking.

1 ¼ cup of non-dairy milk

1 Tbsp grapeseed oil or melted coconut oil

1 tsp vanilla extract

English Muffins

Makes 8 muffins

1 packet yeast

½ cup warm water

1 Tbsp raw honey

½ cup white teff flour

½ cup millet flour

½ cup gluten free oat flour

½ cup tapioca flour

½ cup potato starch

½ tsp xanthan gum

2 tsp baking powder

2 tsp baking soda

½ tsp sea salt

1 cup warm non-dairy milk

2 Tbsp avocado oil

Organic cornmeal

In mixing bowl, warm ½ cup water to 120° F and stir in yeast and honey. Set aside to proof for 5 minutes.

In small bowl whisk together flours, xanthan gum, baking powder, baking soda, and salt. Pour the warm milk and oil into the flour blend using a hand mixer on low speed. Add in the yeast mixture and mix until combined. Set the bowl aside in a warm area and allow to rise for 45 minutes.

Preheat the oven to 325°F degrees. Spray English muffin rings with oil.

Sprinkle baking sheet lined with parchment with cornmeal. Place muffin rings on the baking sheet. Using a scoop, add muffin mixture to the rings and sprinkle with cornmeal. Bake for 15 minutes, then flip and bake 15 minutes more until golden brown. Cool completely.

Blueberry Breakfast Burgers

Serves 4

Burgers for breakfast? Absolutely! Especially with this hearty blend of breakfast flavors that will fill your belly and lift your spirits for the day. These are rich in fiber, protein and are mouthwatering.

2 cups chickpeas, cooked and mashed

½ cup gluten free rolled oats

3 Tbsp almond butter

2 Tbsp maple syrup

¼ tsp sea salt

½ tsp cinnamon

1 cup blueberries

2 Tbsp coconut oil

Combine the chickpeas, oats, almond butter, maple syrup, sea salt and cinnamon in a food processor and pulse until combined. Add blueberries and pulse 3 to 4 times. Form into patties.

Heat oil in a skillet over medium high heat. Add patties and cook until browned on both sides.

Vegan Southwest Scramble

Serves 4

I used to like an egg scramble and found that I missed them terribly when I gave up eggs. Since I try to avoid soy products, I was thrilled when I found hemp tofu. I created this dish to meet my desire for a healthy southwest breakfast free from common allergens.

2 tsp extra virgin olive oil, divided

2 packages hempseed tofu, rinsed, patted dry and crumbled

1 tsp ground cumin

1½ tsp chili powder

½ tsp turmeric powder

½ tsp sea salt, divided

¼ cup chopped red bell pepper

1 small organic zucchini, diced

¾ cup frozen organic corn, thawed

4 organic scallions, sliced

½ cup black beans, drained and rinsed

½ cup pico de gallo

¼ cup chopped fresh cilantro

Heat one teaspoon of the olive oil in a large nonstick skillet over medium heat. Add tofu, cumin, chili powder, turmeric and ¼ tsp sea salt and cook, stirring occasionally, until the tofu begins to brown, 4 to 6 minutes. Transfer to a bowl.

Add the remaining oil to the pan. Add pepper, zucchini, corn, scallions and the remaining ¼ tsp salt. Cook, stirring, until the vegetables are just tender, about 3 minutes. Stir in the black beans and sauté until warmed through. Return the tofu to the pan and cook about 2 minutes more. Remove from the heat and top each serving with 2 Tbsp pico de gallo and 1 Tbsp cilantro.

Fabulous Fiber Bread

Makes 1 loaf (approximately 10 slices)

This bread is free from many of the common allergens and is yeast-free. It is a whole grain bread so it has a more dense texture that is reminiscent of the breads you often find in Europe. For this reason, I suggest slicing the bread thinly and toasting it to prevent crumbling. It does utilize a wide array of flours only because it results in better taste and texture. It also enhances the nutritional value and is perfect for the morning slice of toast with fresh jam.

Dry Ingredients:

½ cup brown rice flour

½ cup gluten free oat flour

¼ cup tapioca flour

¼ cup coconut flour

¼ cup ground chia seed

¼ cup almond or hazelnut flour (for nut free version use millet flour)

¼ arrowroot flour

1 tsp guar gum

1 tsp baking soda

1 Tbsp baking powder

½ tsp sea salt

1 tsp apple cider vinegar

1 Tbsp blackstrap molasses or yacon syrup

2 Tbsp raw honey (use coconut nectar for a vegan version)

1 cup warm water mixed with 2 tsp vegan plain gelatin

1 Tbsp coconut oil, melted

½-1 cup warm water

Combine all dry ingredients in large mixer bowl and incorporate well. Add in vinegar, molasses, honey, gelatin mix, coconut oil and water. Turn mixture to medium low speed to fully combine. Pour into greased bread loaf pan and bake at 360° F for 60 minutes.

Breakfast Stuffed Sweet Potato

Serves 1

This is one of my go-to meals when the blustery winter days arrive. The beautiful bright colors of the components in this sweet treat always makes me smile and anticipate the warmer days to come. This is a power packed, nutrient-rich breakfast dish that keeps you full for hours. Scrumptious!

1 small sweet potato, baked

2 Tbsp almond milk

1 Tbsp almond or pecan butter

½ tsp ground cinnamon

1 packet stevia

Pinch sea salt

1 tsp vanilla extract

¼ cup cooked quinoa (I like to cook mine in apple cider for extra flavor)

¼ cup chopped steamed kale

2 Tbsp fresh blueberries

2 tsp maple syrup

Combine almond milk, almond butter, cinnamon, stevia and sea salt in small saucepan and heat to a simmer. Remove from heat and stir in vanilla extract. Pour over sliced sweet potato and top with cooked quinoa, kale and blueberries. Drizzle with maple syrup.

Eggless Omelet

Serves 4

If you can't eat eggs, you don't have to forego a tasty egg-like omelet. This omelet is cooked like a pancake but has all the satisfaction and protein of an omelet, except this one is vegan. Enjoy it with your favorite omelet fillings and toppings!

1 cup chickpea flour

4 Tbsp nutritional yeast flakes

2 Tbsp raw tahini paste

1 tsp baking powder

½ tsp turmeric

Pinch paprika

1 cup water

½ tsp sea salt

½ tsp white pepper

Blend all ingredients in blender until smooth. Stir in filling ingredients. Cook in a nonstick skillet over medium heat until bubbles appear. Flip and cook until set.

Sarah's Favorite Filling:

¼ cup red bell peppers, diced

¼ cup sliced mushrooms

¼ cup chopped artichoke hearts, drained

¼ cup scallions, trimmed and chopped

¼ cup chopped baby spinach

Fresh tarragon

Banana Bread

Makes 2 – 8.5" x 4.5" loaves- 12 servings

This mouth-watering whole grain quick bread is full of fiber and potassium. Kids are drawn to the natural sweetness of the banana and adults appreciate that kids love this nutritious breakfast delight.

½ cup superfine brown rice

½ cup sorghum flour

¾ cup teff flour

½ cup arrowroot

½ cup tapioca flour

¼ cup coconut flour

¾ cup organic brown sugar

1 Tbsp baking powder

1 tsp xanthan gum

1 tsp baking soda

½ tsp sea salt

2 cups mashed ripe bananas (approximately 4 large bananas)

⅔ cup unsweetened non-dairy milk

⅓ cup melted virgin coconut oil

2 Tbsp chia seed mixed with 6 Tbsp warm water

1 Tbsp vanilla

½ tsp ground cinnamon

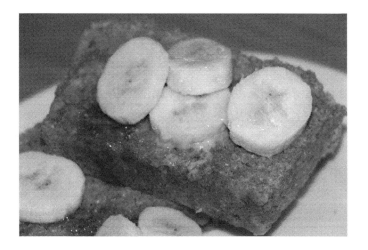

Preheat oven to 375°F.

In a large bowl combine the flours, brown sugar, baking powder, xanthan gum, baking soda and sea salt. Mix well.

Blend bananas in food processor or blender until smooth. Add the non-dairy milk, coconut oil, chia mixture, vanilla, and cinnamon. Pour this mixture into the dry and stir until fully incorporated.

Pour batter into greased loaf pans and bake for 45 minutes or until toothpick comes out clean.

Banana Honey Molasses Muffins

Makes 18 standard size muffins

My mom used to make honey banana muffins for us growing up and the memory was motivating me to create this recipe. I use a combination of molasses and honey for an extra rich taste and increased iron content. I also add applesauce in addition to the banana so that the muffins are moist. My son loves these and I am certain you will too!

4 mashed small bananas (about 2 cups mashed)

½ cup coconut palm sugar

½ cup applesauce

6 Tbsp melted coconut oil

6 Tbsp raw honey

2 Tbsp molasses (not blackstrap)

1 Tbsp vanilla extract

1 tsp apple cider vinegar

Dry Ingredients:

2 cups Sarah's all purpose flour blend

½ cup gluten free oat flour

½ cup almond flour

2 tsp baking powder

1 tsp baking soda

½ tsp sea salt

½ tsp cinnamon

Preheat oven to 350°F.

Grease and flour two muffin pans or use paper liners. Set aside.

In a large bowl, using a hand mixer, combine bananas, sugar, applesauce, oil, honey, molasses, vanilla extract and vinegar. On low speed, add the dry ingredients, a little at a time until well blended. Fill muffin cups about two thirds full.

Bake for 20 to 25 minutes or until a toothpick inserted in the center comes out dry and clean. Allow to cool for 10 to 15 minutes before serving.

Protein Pancakes

Makes 1 Serving

Pancakes do not have to be unhealthy or be high in refined carbohydrates. These protein pancakes are protein rich and are packed with fiber and flavor. This recipe makes a very generous portion so savor every bite guilt free because they are nutritious and low in sugar. This breakfast will build muscle while slimming your waistline. These pancakes freeze well by separating cooled pancakes with parchment paper and placing inside a freezer bag. Please note that it is important to cook these slowly over low heat as the protein powder may cause the pancake to brown more quickly.

1 scoop vegan protein powder

3 Tbsp uncooked gluten free rolled oats

1 Tbsp Sarah's pancake mix flour blend (see Extras)

1 Tbsp applesauce

2 tsp melted coconut oil

2 oz. non-dairy milk

⅛ tsp baking powder

⅛ tsp baking soda

1 tsp gluten free maple extract

1 large egg, whisked or egg replacer for 1 egg

1 Tbsp coconut palm sugar or 1 packet stevia (optional)

Combine all ingredients except fruit in a bowl. Heat a non-stick griddle over low heat. Ladle pancake mixture onto pan and allow to brown, flipping over once bubbles form (about 3 to 4 minutes). Cook on the other side until set. Serve topped with berries, fruit juice sweetened jam, sunflower seed butter or pure maple syrup if desired.

Superfood Sunrise Bars

Makes 8 bars

This granola bar is designed for those individuals seeking to boost energy. The bars are full of anti-oxidants, healthy fats and protein and are a wonderful pre- or post-workout snack.

1 cup organic gluten free rolled oats

¼ cup dried goji berries, soaked for 1 hour

½ cup medjool dates, pitted

½ cup almond butter

½ cup vegan protein powder

½ cup unsweetened applesauce

¼ cup organic unrefined coconut oil, melted

2 tsp maca powder

1 tsp organic vanilla extract

1 pinch sea salt

2 Tbsp shredded coconut

Preheat oven to 350°F.

Mix all ingredients together except coconut in food processor. Press into baking dish and sprinkle with coconut. Bake for 30 minutes or until edges are golden. Allow to cool before cutting into squares.

Maple Raspberry Scones

Makes 6 large or 12 small scones

Nearby my grandparents' house there was a bakery we visited to purchase our favorite baked treats. I always grabbed a bag of scones to take home and although these are not cinnamon, I love the mouth feel. My scones are a perfect cross between a muffin and a biscuit and are not too heavy.

1 ½ cups sorghum flour

½ cup tapioca flour

1 Tbsp baking powder

¾ tsp xanthan gum

½ tsp sea salt

½ cup Spectrum butter flavored vegetable shortening

⅓ cup maple syrup

½ cup + 2 Tbsp cold non-dairy milk

1 Tbsp vanilla extract

1 heaping cup fresh organic raspberries

Preheat oven to 425°F.

Place the flours, baking powder, xanthan gum, and sea salt into a medium mixing bowl and whisk together well. Cut in the shortening with your fingers or a pastry cutter until coarse crumbs are formed.

In a separate small bowl whisk together the maple syrup, non-dairy milk, and vanilla extract. Add to the dry ingredients and quickly mix together with a fork or wooden spoon until the dough thickens. Fold in the raspberries, being very careful not to over mix. The dough will be thick.

Drop by the large spoonful onto a greased cookie sheet or in a non-stick scone pan and bake for about 15 to 17 minutes for small scones or 20 to 22 minutes for large scones.

Breakfast Brown Rice

Serves 4

The morning bowl of oatmeal can become mundane when eaten every day. It is extremely important for us to not eat the same foods everyday so that we can maximize nutrition. Using brown rice is a nutritious and gratifying way to start your day and is easily found at any grocery store. This recipe is also a fantastic way to use up your leftover brown rice from chinese food takeout.

2 cups cooked brown rice

1 cup canned coconut milk

2 tsp cinnamon

Pinch sea salt

2 tsp gluten free maple extract

2 Tbsp chopped walnuts

2 Tbsp fruit juice sweetened dried cranberries

1 packet stevia or 1 dropperful English Toffee liquid stevia

Place cooked brown rice in medium pot over medium high heat. Add coconut milk, cinnamon, and sea salt and bring to a light boil. Reduce heat and simmer for 10 to 15 minutes. Remove from heat and stir in maple extract, walnuts, cranberries, and stevia. Serve warm or cold.

Applesauce Muffins

Makes 12 standard muffins

This was my grandmother's recipe that originally had walnuts studded throughout the bread. Since my nephew has a nut allergy, I thought it would be nice to still share tradition with him without danger. This one's for you Evan!

Wet ingredients:

1 cup applesauce

½ cup coconut palm sugar

¼ cup maple syrup

¼ cup avocado oil

¼ cup coconut milk mixed with ½ tsp apple cider vinegar

2 Tbsp ground chia seed mixed with 6 Tbsp warm water

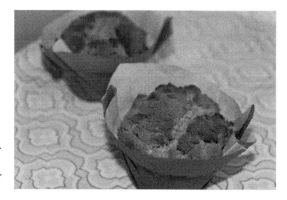

Dry ingredients:

½ cups Sarah's all purpose flour blend

½ cup gluten free oat flour

1 Tbsp baking powder

1 tsp cinnamon

¼ tsp sea salt

¼ tsp nutmeg

Topping:

2 Tbsp brown sugar

2 Tbsp almond meal or gluten free quick oats

2 Tbsp melted Earth Balance soy free spread

½ tsp cinnamon

Preheat oven to 350°F.

Mix topping ingredients in a bowl.

In a large mixing bowl, whisk together the wet ingredients. Next, add the dry ingredients and stir until thoroughly combined. Scoop into muffin tins (dough will be slightly sticky) and sprinkle with topping mixture. Bake for 25 to 30 minutes or until toothpick comes out clean.

Breakfast Butternut Bowl

Serves 3

Soup for breakfast? Absolutely! This soup is thick, creamy and so rich that even the most discriminating palate would not imagine this blend is dairy free. Try this simple and tasty soup at your next family gathering if you seek to impress a crowd.

4 cups butternut squash

2 cups heated vegetable stock

3 Tbsp maple syrup

¾ tsp minced fresh ginger

3 oz. canned coconut cream

Pinch ground nutmeg

Sea salt and pepper to taste

Plain unsweetened coconut milk yogurt, garnish, optional

Pumpkin seeds, garnish

Roast butternut squash in oven for 30 to 40 minutes at 400° F. Meanwhile, gently heat vegetable stock in pot over low heat. When squash is slightly browned, add all ingredients into a bowl and puree with a stick blender. Stir in the coconut cream and season with salt, pepper, and nutmeg.

Top with a dollop of unsweetened coconut milk yogurt and pumpkin seeds.

Note: This soup is also delicious when blended with 1 scoop of vegan protein powder per 2 cup serving and sprinkled with Sarah's granola.

Sarah's Granola

Makes 8 servings

I am including this recipe in honor of one of my dearest friends, Erica, who always is grateful for the gift of granola. She is ecstatic whenever I offer her a batch of granola and I fancy making it for my loved ones. It is perfect in so many ways- sweet, crunchy, and nutty. I suggest eating it topped with fresh Cashew Milk (see Beverages).

3 cups gluten free rolled oats

1 cup slivered almonds or nuts of choice other

½ cup shredded coconut (optional)

¼ cup dark brown sugar

1 tsp cinnamon

½ tsp sea salt

¼ cup melted coconut oil

2 Tbsp maple syrup

1 tsp vanilla extract

1 cup raisins, cranberries or mixture of dried fruit

Preheat oven to 250°F.

In a large bowl combine oats, nuts, coconut, brown sugar, cinnamon, and sea salt. Mix well. In a separate bowl combine oil, maple syrup, and vanilla. Pour the oil blend into the oat mixture and stir until thoroughly blended. Pour onto two parchment-lined cookie sheets and bake for about 45 minutes, stirring every 15 minutes for even cooking. Remove from oven, stir in dried fruit, and allow to cool for an hour before serving.

Pops' Blueberry Muffins

Makes 12 standard size muffins

My grandfather used to make these delectable muffins that were light, delicate and slightly sweet. I made a few modifications over the years and have made them vegan and gluten free. They are just as good as the fond memories of the love I have for my grandfather.

Wet ingredients:

½ cup coconut palm sugar

¼ cup organic sugar

⅓ cup Earth Balance soy free spread

¼ cup applesauce

½ cup almond milk mixed with 1 tsp apple cider vinegar and 1 tsp vanilla extract

Dry ingredients:

1 ½ cups Sarah's all purpose flour blend

½ cup gluten free oat flour

1 Tbsp baking powder

½ tsp baking soda

½ tsp sea salt

Pinch xanthan gum

2 cups blueberries

Cinnamon sugar

Preheat oven to 375°F.

Cream the sugars and Earth Balance until creamy. Add the applesauce and beat well. In a separate bowl, combine dry ingredients whisking to mix thoroughly. Toss the blueberries into the dry mixture. Slowly stir in the wet ingredients, one third at a time alternating with the almond milk mixture.

Scoop into muffin cups and sprinkle with cinnamon sugar. Bake for 30 minutes or until muffins are golden and a toothpick comes out clean.

Yeast Free Egg Bread

Makes 10 slices

Although this bread is very simple, it is quite tasty and a real treat for those who are trying to avoid yeasted products. It is scrumptious with a smear of avocado, tomato and sprouts with a dab of grainy Dijon mustard.

<u>Wet Ingredients:</u>

3 large eggs, whisked

¼ cup ground chia seeds

2 tsp apple cider vinegar

2 Tbsp avocado oil

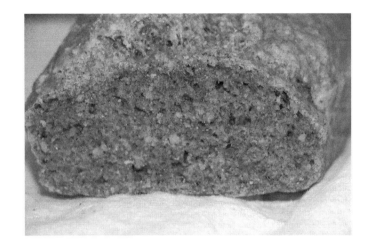

<u>Dry Ingredients:</u>

½ cup almond flour

½ cup gluten free oat flour

¼ cup tapioca starch

1 tsp baking soda

¼ tsp sea salt

Preheat oven to 350°F.

In a large bowl, blend the eggs, ground chia seeds, vinegar, and oil with a hand mixer until smooth. Add the dry ingredients and mix until dough gets thick. Pour dough into a greased small loaf pan and bake for 30 to 35 minutes, or until a toothpick comes out clean. Cool before slicing.

Chocolate Chip Scones

Makes 8 scones

Scones are a wonderful treat for a weekend breakfast and although they may seem like an unhealthy choice, these are made from whole grains. These should not be an everyday breakfast but I find them to be a wonderful birthday breakfast for the munchkins in your life. I also have found that once they become stale, they make fantastic homemade breadcrumbs for coating chicken, fish and tofu.

1 ½ cups Sarah's All Purpose Flour Blend

½ cup gluten free oat flour

2 tsp baking powder

½ tsp baking soda

¼ tsp sea salt

½ cup Earth Balance soy free spread

½ cup vegan dark chocolate chips

1 tsp vanilla

¾ cup almond milk mixed with 1 Tbsp apple cider vinegar

Preheat oven to 400°F.

In a large bowl, whisk the flours, baking powder, baking soda and sea salt. Add the Earth Balance and use a pastry blender to blend into a coarse meal. Add the chocolate chips, then stir in vanilla and almond milk mixture.

Bake in a greased scone pan for 15 minutes or until golden brown and a toothpick comes out clean.

BEVERAGES

Cashew Milk

Makes 5 cups

Making your own nut milks at home takes less time than you would imagine. In addition, by blending up your own milk at home, there is no need to add unnecessary oils and stabilizers to the mix. Cashew milk is extremely creamy, and is a favorite among kids, especially blended with freeze-dried strawberry powder.

1 cup cashews

3 - 4 cups water

2 pitted dates (if desired)

1 tsp vanilla (if desired)

Blend all ingredients in high speed blender until creamy and smooth. Store in fridge for up to one week.

Juices

All recipes serve 1 and are best prepared using a juicer

Here are a few recipes for my favorite juices, especially after the holidays when I want to clean all of the nasty toxins out of my system and increase my metabolic rate. These juices also make for an energizing late afternoon quaff.

"The Regular"

1 head romaine

1 carrot

½ cucumber

2 stalks celery

1 cup spinach or kale

1 lemon, peeled

1 lime, peeled

Very Vegetabilcious

2 large carrots

3 stalks celery

½ cup parsley

4 large spinach leaves

¼ beet

½ cup alfalfa sprouts

Energy Booster

1 small sweet potato

¼ beet

1 clove garlic

1 lime, peeled

1 grapefruit, juiced

1 celery stalk

½" slice of fresh ginger

Orange Sunshine

2 pears

3 pink grapefruits, peeled

1 sweet potato

Chocolate "Milk"

2 heads romaine

5 carrots

2 Tbsp raw cacao

1 tsp lucuma powder

1 dropperful liquid chocolate stevia

Run the romaine and carrots through a juicer. Stir in raw cacao, lucuma, and stevia until well combined.

Smoothies

All recipes serve 1

I drink a smoothie almost every morning because they are easy and portable. More importantly, I find that drinking a smoothie in the morning is the best breakfast to placate my hunger and energize me until lunch hour. My smoothie recipes are designed to give you extra energy, increased focus, and provide a properly balanced breakfast or snack. And, kids love them!

For all recipes, add 1 to 2 cups of ice and blend in a high speed blender until smooth.

Cinnamon Roll Smoothie

1 ½ cups unsweetened almond milk

1 frozen banana

1 Tbsp raw cashew butter

1 tsp sesame seeds

1 tsp ground cinnamon

1 tsp vanilla extract

Pinch of sea salt

2 pitted medjool dates

Green Nutty Chimp

1 frozen banana

2 Tbsp almond butter

½ cup raw spinach

1 cup unsweetened almond milk

1 scoop vanilla vegan protein powder

Energy Booster

½ cup frozen banana

½ cup pineapple

½ cup coconut water

1 tsp local bee pollen

1 tsp hempseed oil

1 cup coconut water

1 scoop vegan protein powder

Almond Butter Cup Smoothie

¼ cup organic gluten free old fashioned oats

½ cup coconut water

½ cup unsweetened almond milk

2 pitted medjool dates

½ banana

2 Tbsp almond butter

2 Tbsp cocoa powder

1 tsp vanilla extract

1 scoop vegan protein powder (if desired)

Frozen Mocha Maca Latte

Serves 1

Even people I know who hate coffee love this frothy treat. It is light, creamy and free of the bitter aftertaste sometimes found in coffee drinks. It tastes similar to coffee ice cream.

1 cup cashew milk

¼ cup filtered water or cooled reishi mushroom tea

1 pitted date

1 Tbsp raw cacao

2 tsp maca powder

½ tsp mesquite powder

1 tsp vanilla

½ frozen banana

1 tsp high quality espresso powder

Ice

Combine all ingredients in high speed blender and run until smooth and creamy.

Pregnancy Protein Shake

Serves 1

I realize not everyone is pregnant, however this protein shake is full of essential nutrients critical for proper cell development including calcium, selenium, folate and vitamin E. Even if you aren't expecting a baby, you can expect a lovely and refreshing treat.

1 cup cashew milk

4 oz. plain unsweetened coconut milk yogurt

4 oz. raspberry leaf tea

½ cup of your favorite berries (frozen or seasonal)

½ small banana

¼ avocado

1 scoop of vegan protein powder

1 handful raw kale or spinach

1 Tbsp almond butter

1 Tbsp raw honey

1 Brazil nut

Combine all ingredients in blender and run on high speed until smooth.

Pumpkin Pie Latte

Makes 1 latte (16 oz.)

It is easy to fall in love with this warm mug of pumpkin bliss during the bitter days of Autumn. Even children love this- just subsitute warm apple cider for the coffee. Perfectly pumpkin!

1 cup almond milk

¼ cup canned pumpkin

½ tsp vanilla extract

Maple syrup or stevia to taste

½ tsp pumpkin pie spice

1 cup hot coffee

Pinch sea salt

Combine the almond milk and canned pumpkin in sauce pan, and bring to a simmer. Remove from heat and whisk in vanilla, sweetener and spices. Pour ½ of the mixture into mug and top with coffee. With electric whisk or frother, mix the remaining milk/pumpkin mix until frothy. Pour over coffee and sprinkle with sea salt.

Anemia Buster Blend

Serves 1

If you are feeling weak and tired, this is the beverage for you. Not only is it delicious, it delivers powerful nutrients to every cell in the body at lightning speed. Feel free to add some fresh beet juice for extra oomph in building the red blood cells.

1 cup organic baby spinach

1 cup fresh almond milk

1 tsp spirulina powder

½ peeled grapefruit

1 handful fresh mint

1 oz. pumpkin seeds

2 Tbsp organic raisins

1" grated ginger

1 tsp raw honey

1 cup lemon juice

Combine all ingredients in a blender and blend until completely smooth.

Holiday Nog

Serves 4

As a child I remember sipping small cups of egg nog. When I gave up dairy, I never found the dairy free versions to taste good. I devised this incredibly rich nog to resemble the traditional nog so that your guests would never guess it is an imposter.

2 cups cashew creamer (recipe follows)

2 packets pure stevia

1 tsp gluten free maple syrup extract

1 tsp organic extra virgin coconut oil

1 tsp rum extract

1 tsp vanilla extract

½ tsp fresh grated nutmeg, plus additional for

1 frozen large banana

Ground cinnamon, for garnish, if desired

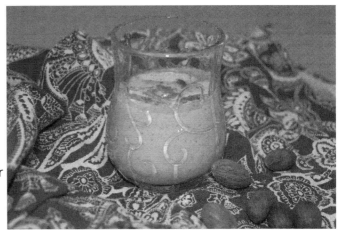

Add all ingredients to high speed blender and run until smooth. Add ice if desired. Sprinkle with cinnamon when serving, if desired.

Cashew Creamer:

1 cup raw cashews

2 cups water

2 dates, pitted

½ tsp vanilla extract

Pour the nuts and water in a high speed blender and blend well. Add the dates and vanilla and blend until silky smooth.

Hot Cocoa Mix

Makes approximately 16 servings

Hot cocoa mixes are loaded with refined sugar, low quality cocoa, ultra pasturized milk powders and unnatural fillers. This mix is pure, simple, low calorie and a must have in your pantry. It is also a great base for ice cream (in case you happen to have leftover when the warm weather arrives).

1 cup organic high quality cocoa powder (Guittard, etc.)

½ cup organic powdered sugar

3 packets pure stevia extract

½ cup allergen free vegan mini chocolate chips

1 Tbsp organic cornstarch (optional)

¼ tsp sea salt

Combine all ingredients in a large glass jar. Replace the lid and shake to combine. Keep stored in your pantry for up to 9 months or in fridge or freezer for up to 14 months.

Hot Cocoa Preparation instructions:

Mix two tablespoons of cocoa mix with eight ounces warmed non-dairy milk of choice.

Richest Hot Sipping Chocolate

Makes 2 servings

The name of this recipe says it best. I have been known to have a mild addiction to hot cocoa and this is an extra decadent sipping chocolate that I enjoy the most. Adding peppermint oil and a candy cane for stirring is another favorite, especially on Christmas Eve while waiting for Santa. It is thick, creamy and sinful. YUM!

1 (14 oz.) can coconut milk

1 tsp vanilla bean

1 tsp vanilla extract

¾ cup chopped semisweet chocolate

1 Tbsp organic brown sugar

In a 2-quart pan, warm milk and vanilla bean over low heat to blend flavors, stirring often; do not boil. Add chopped chocolate to hot milk; stir over low heat until chocolate melts. Remove from heat and stir in vanilla extract. Pour hot chocolate into mugs and serve with Whipped Cream (see Extras) or vegan marshmallows.

Dreamy Creamy Orange Shake

Serves 1

When summer rolls around, I sometimes miss the Push Pops from the ice cream truck. For a very long time I felt deprived, so a friend and I created this treat with the delightful orange treat in mind. Our version is rich, creamy, cool and so delicious! It is a perfect ending to a day by the pool.

1 medium frozen orange

¼ frozen avocado

¼ large frozen banana

2 Tbsp coconut cream (from full-fat canned coconut milk)

1 cup almond milk

1 Tbsp lucuma powder

¼ tsp vanilla

1 date, pitted

Zest of an orange

Place all ingredients into a blender and blend until smooth.

SNACKS

Grain Free Crackers

Makes 24 - 1" crackers

This is a savory cracker that you can vary according to your taste preferences. I like to use a garlic herb blend, however feel free to substitute whatever flavors you like. For example, a Mexican or Indian spice blend will result in a very tasty cracker.

½ cup almond flour

¼ cup sorghum flour

2 Tbsp ground chia seed

2 Tbsp sorghum bran

½ tsp baking powder

½ cup almond milk

1 Tbsp raw honey

1 Tbsp garlic herb seasoning

½ tsp sea salt

Preheat oven to 350 °F.

In a large bowl, stir together almond flour, sorghum flour, chia seed, sorghum bran and baking powder until well combined. Add almond milk, honey, spices and sea salt. Roll out to ¼" thickness between 2 sheets of waxed paper. Transfer to a parchment lined cookie sheet and cut into slices. Bake until golden brown (about 30 minutes).

Homemade Dill Pickles

Makes 5 pints

I wanted to include this recipe because making your own pickles is ridiculously easy and requires little time in the kitchen. You will be extremely surprised how crunchy and delicious pickles are when you make them at home. I created this recipe because I love pickles but hate that many varieties use white vinegar and beet sugar, which is often GMO, and I wanted a "clean" version. I hope you will find these crispy slices as pleasing as I do.

3 Tbsp pickling spice

4 cups raw apple cider vinegar

4 cups water

¼ cup organic sugar

¼ cup coconut palm sugar

½ cup sea salt

5 bay leaves

5 cloves garlic

2 ½ tsp mustard seeds

5 heads fresh dill

14 cups sliced pickling cucumbers (¼" lengthwise slices)

5 (16 oz.) pint glass preserving jars with lids and bands

Prepare boiling water canner. Heat jars and lids in simmering water until ready for use. Do not boil. Set bands aside.

Place pickling spice in a mesh teabag and tie with culinary twine. Combine the pickling spice, vinegar, water, sugars, and sea salt and spice bag in a large stainless steel saucepan. Bring to a boil over medium-high heat. Reduce heat and boil gently for 15 minutes.

Place 1 bay leaf, 1 garlic clove, ½ tsp mustard seeds and 1 head of dill into each jar. Pack cucumber slices into hot jars leaving ½" headspace and ladle hot pickling liquid into jar to cover cucumbers leaving ½" headspace. Wipe rim and screw on bands tightly.

Process in a boiling water canner for 15 minutes. Remove jars and cool. Store in pantry for up to 1 year.

Pretzels

Makes 8 pretzels

I was known to indulge in the giant soft pretzels while in Manhattan or at a sporting event. After going gluten free, it was challenge for me not to succumb and risk being inflamed for weeks when presented with a doughy pretzel topped with kosher salt and yellow mustard. Fortunately, this recipe erased the temptation. These are much crunchier but so good!

¼ cup baking soda

2 ½ cups seltzer water

½ cup brown rice flour

½ cup tapioca flour

¼ cup gluten free oat flour

¼ potato starch

½ tsp baking soda

½ cup almond or coconut milk plus ½ Tbsp apple cider vinegar

2 Tbsp yacon syrup or raw honey

1 Tbsp sea salt flakes, for topping

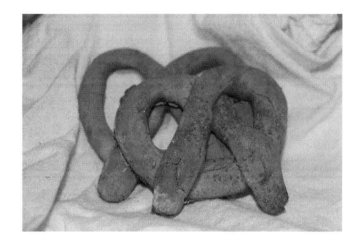

In a stock pot, dissolve ¼ cup baking soda in 2 ½ cups seltzer water. Bring water to a boil, and then remove from heat. Preheat oven to 375°F.

In a large bowl, sift together the brown rice flour, tapioca flour, gluten free oat flour, potato starch, and baking soda. Stir in milk substitute and yacon and mix until dough pulls together. Turn dough out onto a lightly floured surface, and knead briefly to thoroughly blend ingredients.

Divide dough into 8 equal pieces. Roll each piece into a cylinder approximately 12 inches long. Form into classic pretzel shape. Pinch ends to seal. Place on lightly greased cookie sheets. Brush pretzels with baking soda solution.

Sprinkle pretzels with flaked salt, and bake in preheated oven about 8 minutes or until golden brown.

Caramel Coconut Kale Chips

Serves 3

These are not your standard kale chips because this is a sweet version. These make for an iron-packed dessert when I am craving crunchy sweetness. Nobody can resist the crunch and caramel goodness of these chips.

1 bunch kale

1 avocado

½ Cashew Milk (see beverages)

¼ cup lucuma powder

1 tsp vanilla

¼ cup raw honey

1 Tbsp organic brown sugar

1 dropperful vanilla stevia

2 Tbsp coconut butter

Wash kale pieces and dry. Chop into pieces.

Meanwhile, place remaining ingredients in blender and blend until smooth. Pour over kale and massage with hands until well coated. Spread onto a teflex sheet and dehydrate at 115°F for 24 hours or until crunchy, flipping every few hours to ensure crunch.

When completely cooled, store in an airtight bag for up to 2 weeks for maximum freshness.

Cheesy Kale Chips

Serves 6

Here is another delicious kale chip recipe that I make on a regular basis. Similar versions are available in stores however I find the prices to be outrageous for something so easy to make at home. I hope you enjoy them as much as I do.

2 bunches of kale, washed, dried, stems removed and torn into medium sized pieces

1 cup cashews, soaked for 2 hours

2 Tbsp lemon juice

¼ cup nutritional yeast

¼ cup red bell pepper

1 tsp black pepper

½ tsp sea salt

Pinch of cayenne pepper

Put all ingredients except the kale into a high speed blender and process until you achieve a smooth consistency. Pour the mixture into a large bowl and add kale. Massage the liquid into the kale with hands until kale softens.

Spread kale onto a teflex sheet and bake in a dehydrator at 115°F for 24 hours or until crunchy, flipping once half way through.

When completely cooled, store in an airtight bag for up to 2 weeks for maximum freshness.

Fresh Salsa

Serves 8

Many salsas contain unnecessary ingredients including fillers, preservatives, sugar and/or vinegar. This recipe is more flavorful than the store bought versions, is low in sodium and sugar free.

1 – 15 oz. can diced tomatoes, no salt added

1 – 15 oz. can fire roasted diced tomatoes with chilies

1 jalapeno pepper, diced (wear gloves!)

1 small onion, diced

2 cloves garlic, minced

¼ cup chopped fresh cilantro

½ tsp ground cumin

1-2 Tbsp fresh lime juice

¼ tsp black pepper

Sea salt to taste

Combine all ingredients in a bowl and serve with organic tortilla chips.

Guacamole

Serves 8

Although making guacamole takes a little bit of time, it is worth the effort! You can add your own quirky twists like I do, sometimes adding pomegranate seeds, fresh mango, pumpkins seeds or even coconut. Allow your creative side to contribute to the process and you will be surprised at the culinary treasures you concoct.

4 avocados, pitted

1 small tomato, finely diced

¼ cup onion, finely chopped

1 clove garlic, minced

1 small jalapeno, seeded and minced

Juice of ½ lime

2 Tbsp fresh cilantro, chopped (optional)

Celtic sea salt and black pepper to taste

Mash avocados until chunky. Add in remaining ingredients and stir until combined and desired consistency.

Roasted Red Pepper Hummus

Serves 4-6

Who doesn't like hummus? I know a few people who swear they hate it, but yet they always are munching on my red pepper hummus when they stop by for a visit. Not all hummus is created equal and making your own ensures you can control the ingredients, resulting in a fresh and fantastic spread.

1 - 15 oz. can garbanzo beans, drained

1 - 4 oz. jar roasted red peppers

1 Tbsp tahini paste (omit if allergic to sesame or use cashew or hemp seed butter)

Juice of ½ a lemon

1 small clove garlic

½ tsp ground cumin

½ tsp sea salt

1 Tbsp chopped fresh parsley

2-3 Tbsp extra virgin olive oil

Combine beans and red peppers in food processor and process until combined. Next, add the tahini, lemon juice, garlic, and spices and pulse to mix. With motor running, drizzle in the olive oil until desired consistency is achieved. Serve immediately, or store in refrigerator for up to 1 week.

Sunflower Veggie Spread

Serves 4

This recipe is super easy and extremely affordable. It is rich in protein, vitamin C, lycopene and is tasty spread on a slice of the Fabulous Fiber Bread and topped with avocado and sprouts. It is filling and makes for a healthy power-packed meal.

1 cup sunflower seeds, soaked 1 hour or more

½ red bell pepper

1 scallion

3 soaked unsulphured sundried tomatoes

½ large carrot, chopped

1 stalk celery

1 Tbsp coconut aminos

1 Tbsp lemon juice

1 tsp cumin

1 tsp sea salt

½ tsp black pepper

2 Tbsp water

Blend all ingredients except the spices and water in a food processor until it begins to form a paste. Drizzle in the water until it reaches a consistency you like. Add the spices, adding more to taste. Serve with the Fabulous Fiber Bread or Grain Free Crackers.

Steamy Broccoli Dip

Serves 8

When football season is in full swing, this dip is certain to make a regular appearance at your potluck events. It is very rich and should be balanced by serving with plenty of low calorie crunchers like celery, carrots, jicama, sugar snap peas or raw asparagus for dipping.

½ cup vegan cream cheese

½ cup avocado mayo (see extras section)

¼ cup nutritional yeast

1 tsp minced garlic

1 ½ tsp sea salt

½ tsp onion powder

¼ cup vegan shredded mozzarella cheese

12 oz. frozen chopped broccoli, thawed and strained of excess liquid

Preheat oven to 400°F.

Combine cream cheese, avocado mayo, nutritional yeast, garlic, sea salt, and onion powder in a food processor and run until smooth. Pulse in cheese and broccoli and scoop into greased baking dish. Bake for 15 to 20 minutes until bubbly. Serve with tortilla chips and lots of fresh vegetables.

Crunchy Chickpea Poppers

Makes 8 servings

Chickpea Poppers are a wonderful high protein snack to carry on-the-go. I urge you to experiment with different seasonings, varying from sweet to savory to find your favorite blend. You can also add these tiny bites to your favorite trail mix for a delightful change.

4 cups canned chickpeas, rinsed and drained
2 Tbsp avocado or coconut oil
1 Tbsp seasoning of your choice

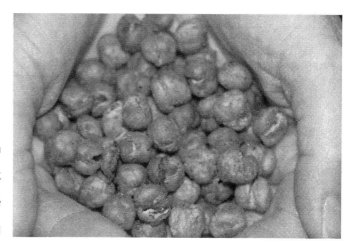

Place rinsed chickpeas in bowl. Drizzle with oil and sprinkle with seasonings (cumin, black pepper, salt, chili powder, paprika, etc.). Place on a baking sheet and bake at 400°F, stirring every 15 minutes, for 45 minutes or until golden. Allow to cool.

Espinaca

Serves 8

I worked at a Mexican restaurant throughout college and this dip was my absolute favorite item on the menu. Unfortunately, I am no longer able to partake in this creamy cheesy dip at restaurants, but I have formulated my own version that meets the craving for cheese dip when it strikes.

16 oz. vegan cream cheese, softened

8 oz. shredded vegan pepper jack cheese

4 oz. frozen spinach, thawed

1 small onion, chopped

1 - 10 oz. can fire roasted diced tomatoes with chilies, drained

1 cup canned light coconut milk

1 tsp miso paste

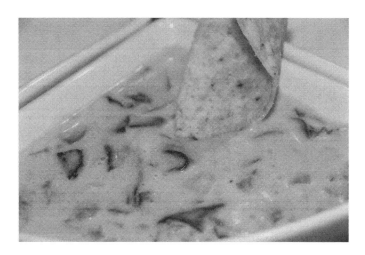

Place thawed spinach in an old towel or a piece of cheesecloth and squeeze out all extra liquid. Next, place all ingredients in crock pot (or on stovetop on the lowest heat) until cheese is fully melted. For a traditional approach, serve with organic corn tortilla chips.

Cranberry Cheese Spread

Serves 8

This appetizer offers a beautiful presentation fitting for any special occasion. And because it is dairy free, it is safe to sit at room temperature.

Cheese:

1 cup cashews, soaked 2 hours

½ cup macadamia nuts, soaked 2 hours

½ cup great northern beans, drained and rinsed

2 Tbsp lemon juice

1 Tbsp orange juice

2 tsp mild miso paste

½ tsp sea salt

Place cheese ingredients in high speed blender or food processor and blend until smooth. Line a bowl with plastic wrap and pour into the bowl. Chill for 4 to 6 hours. Form into a round disc atop a platter, top with compote and serve with gluten free crackers.

Compote:

1 ¼ cup fresh cranberries

½ cup pitted dates, chopped

3 Tbsp fresh grape or orange juice

½ tsp orange zest or 2 drops orange essential oil

Pinch sea salt

Add all ingredients to a food processor and pulse until chunky.

Boobie Bar Lactation Cookies

Makes one dozen cookies

I realize not everybody needs lactation cookies, but these are delicious and safe for the whole family. You can omit the brewer's yeast without changing the texture of the cookies as well. These cookies are packed with B vitamins, protein, and fiber. They are amazing for helping mommies struggling with their milk supply. I suggest eating 2 per day to see a positive change in your milk supply.

¼ cup Earth Balance soy free spread, coconut or avocado oil

½ cup coconut palm sugar

¼ cup organic brown sugar (omit for less sweet cookies)

1 Tbsp vanilla extract

⅓ cup water mixed with 3 Tbsp flaxseed meal

5 Tbsp Brewer's yeast

¼ cup unsweetened applesauce

½ cup almond butter

2 tsp cinnamon

1 ½ tsp baking powder

½ tsp sea salt

½ tsp baking soda

1 ½ cups gluten free old fashioned oats

½ cup additions such as chocolate chips, dried cranberries, raisins, walnuts, etc.

Preheat oven to 350°F.

Using a hand mixer, whip together the Earth Balance, palm sugar, brown sugar, and vanilla. Next add flaxseed blend, brewer's yeast, applesauce, almond butter, cinnamon, baking powder, sea salt, and baking soda. Stir in oats and additions. Using a 2" scooper, scoop dough onto cookies sheet and bake for 12-15 minutes.

Creamy Cinnamon Bean Dip

Serves 6

Dessert hummus!! This sweet hummus is delicious on celery, toast or simply off the spoon! It is also scrumptious atop a baked sweet potato or baked butternut squash.

1 can cannellini beans, drained and rinsed

¼ cup unsweetened plain vegan creamer

2 medjool dates, pitted and soaked

2 Tbsp almond butter

2 tsp raw honey

2 tsp cinnamon

Pinch sea salt

2 Tbsp fruit juice sweetened cranberries

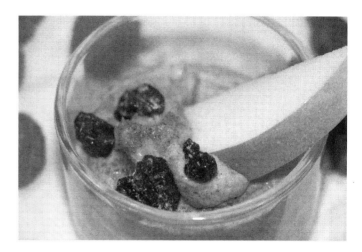

Combine all ingredients except cranberries in food processor and blend well. Top with cranberries and serve.

Chocolate Chip Granola Bars

Makes 16 bars

Who doesn't remember having granola bars in their lunch box as a child? I still walk by the boxes in the stores and wonder why they have been touted as healthy when they are filled with refined ingredients. By making your own bars, you are able to control the flavor and the quality of your ingredients. More importantly, you can drastically reduce the risk of cross contamination by making your portable snack at home. Enjoy!

Nonstick coconut cooking spray

⅓ cup coconut palm sugar

⅓ cup coconut oil

⅓ cup honey

1 cup gluten free quick-cooking oats

¾ cup gluten free old fashioned oats

1 ¼ cups gluten free crispy rice cereal

¼ cup shredded coconut

¼ cup raw pumpkin seeds (optional)

½ tsp sea salt

¼ tsp cinnamon (optional)

½ cup mini gluten free semi-sweet chocolate chips

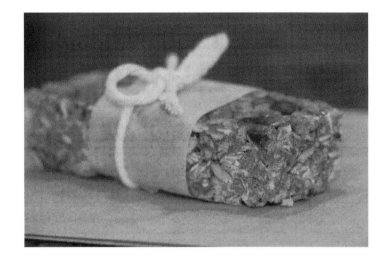

Spray a 9-by-9-inch baking dish with nonstick cooking spray and line with parchment paper. Set aside.

In a saucepan, combine palm sugar, coconut oil, and honey. Place over medium-high heat; bring to a gentle boil. Cook, stirring, for 1 minute. Remove from heat. Cool slightly.

Pour the oats, rice cereal, coconut, pumpkin seeds, sea salt, and spices into a large bowl. Fold in sugar mixture until the mixture is coated and well-combined. Add the chocolate chips and mix. Pour your mixture into the prepared baking dish. Press into dish and set in fridge to cool. Cut into 16 bars and wrap in parchment paper. Store in cool, dark place.

Cocoa Crackers

Makes 16 crackers

These crackers closely resemble chocolate graham crackers, but without the wheat and other potential allergens. I adore these treats and find myself baking a batch regularly because they disappear quickly. Feel free to score the dough into larger pieces so you can enjoy them any way you please. I enjoy them topped with a dollop of almond butter and coconut milk ice cream for a remake on the classic ice cream sandwich.

Dry Ingredients:

½ cup gluten free oat flour

½ cup cocoa powder

¼ cup teff flour

¼ cup almond flour

¼ cup psyllium powder

¼ cup brown sugar or honey powder

2 Tbsp lucuma powder

Wet Ingredients:

2 Tbsp melted coconut oil

1 tsp baking soda

1 ½ tsp baking powder

1 tsp vanilla extract

½ tsp sea salt

¾ cup unsweetened coconut milk

Add all dry ingredients to bowl, and whisk to combine. Add in wet ingredients and blend with hand mixer until dough ball forms. Roll out dough between 2 layers of parchment sprinkled with almond flour to ¼" thickness. Score dough using a pizza cutter into desired cracker size (I like 1" squares). Bake at 350°F for 20 to 25 minutes, rotating once.

Surprising Chocolate Dip/Better Brownie

Serves 6

Dessert hummus is one of my secret indulgences. Your guests will never guess there are beans in this dip and you don't have to share. It can be our little secret…

1 can black beans, drained and rinsed

¼ cup raw cacao powder

2 Tbsp maple syrup

2 packets stevia

¼ tsp sea salt

¼ cup unsweetened coconut creamer

Combine all ingredients in food processor and blend well. Serve topped with chopped nuts, mini vegan chocolate chips or fresh berries for an extra delightful treat.

Note: You can make this into Better Brownies (10 total) by adding:

¼ cup coconut palm sugar

¼ cup vegan chocolate chips

2 Tbsp ground chia seed mixed with 6 Tbsp water

3 Tbsp avocado oil

1 tsp vanilla extract

½ tsp baking powder

½ tsp baking soda

Preheat oven to 350°F.

Blend dip ingredients with brownie additional ingredients with hand mixer. Pour mix into greased loaf pan and bake for 30 minutes. Cool completely before serving.

Sarah's Favorite Crunchy Protein Bars

Makes 16 bars

I prefer to have protein bars handy at all times, especially when traveling. Rather than pay $3 for a specialty protein bar, I make my own bars which allows me to customize the flavors, size, and crunchiness. It also furnishes me control of the quality and freshness of the ingredients.

Cooking spray

1 cup gluten free quick cooking rolled oats

½ cup vegan protein powder

⅓ cup raw sunflower seeds

⅓ cup gluten free oat or rice bran

⅓ cup dried fruit of choice (I like goji berries)

⅓ cup raw slivered almonds

⅓ cup crushed gluten free rice or corn cereal

½ tsp ground cinnamon

3 Tbsp avocado oil or melted coconut oil

2 Tbsp pure maple syrup

2 Tbsp yacon syrup

2 Tbsp mini vegan chocolate chips

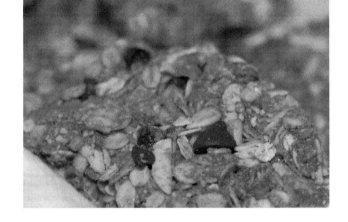

Preheat the oven to 350° F.

Spray a 9 by 9-inch baking pan with cooking spray. Place the oats, protein powder, sunflower seeds, bran, dried fruit, almonds, cereal, and cinnamon in a food processor and pulse until the mixture is finely chopped. Add the oil and syrups and pulse until the mixture is well combined. Stir in chocolate chips. Press into the baking pan making sure it is spread evenly. Bake until just done, about 20 minutes.

Vanilla Bean Chia Seed Pudding

Serves 4

I am jubilant about chia seed pudding. I enjoy it for breakfast, dessert or a quick snack.   It can be made with almond milk and stevia, but I prefer the caramel taste of the dates combined with the cashew milk.

4 cups water

1 cup cashews

2 dates, pitted

2 tsp vanilla extract

Pinch sea salt

Combine all ingredients in a high speed blender until creamy and smooth.

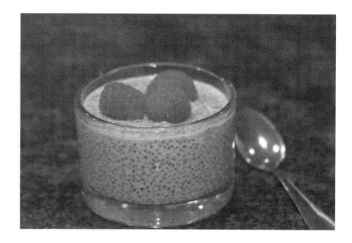

¾ cup chia seeds

¼ cup maple syrup or agave

2 tsp fresh vanilla bean

Stir above ingredients into cashew mixture. Stir well and chill overnight for best results.

Graham Crackers

Makes 24 full-size graham crackers

Graham crackers are a lunchbox necessity for many children. Unfortunately, when following a gluten free diet, a good graham cracker is hard to find. I love to make my own crackers because it is so cost-effective, and I created this recipe to satisfy my graham cracker cravings.

1 cup gluten free oat flour

1 cup Sarah's All Purpose Flour Blend

¼ cup organic cornstarch

¼ cup lucuma powder

1 Tbsp mesquite flour

1 tsp cinnamon

1 tsp baking powder

½ tsp baking soda

½ tsp xanthan gum

½ tsp sea salt

3 Tbsp coconut oil

3 Tbsp Earth Balance soy free spread

5 Tbsp raw honey

¼ cup applesauce

2 tsp vanilla extract

½ cup non-dairy milk

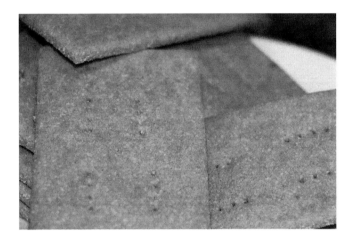

Preheat oven to 350 °F.

In a large bowl, combine flours, cornstarch, lucuma, mesquite, cinnamon, baking powder, baking soda, xanthan gum, and sea salt until combined.

Using a hand mixer, blend the coconut oil, Earth Balance, and honey until smooth. Beat in apple-sauce, vanilla, and non-dairy milk. Gradually add in flours until all are incorporated and continue to mix until dough is formed.

Divide into two sections and pat into disks. Chill each disk for 30 minutes in fridge, and then roll out in between two pieces of parchment paper to ¼" thickness. With knife, score into squares and poke holes in the top with fork. Transfer to parchment lined cookie sheet and bake for 20 minutes, rotating pan halfway through, or until golden. Cool before eating.

Sarah's Vitality Balls

Makes 30 - 1" balls

A quick, healthy and tasty treat for anytime of the day! These are perfect for travel or to keep in the car for easy access. I like to freeze them because they remind me of the frozen candy bars I used to love during my college years.

1 cup gluten free rolled oats

1 cup Cashew Milk (see Beverages)

½ cup raw cacao powder

¼ cup unsweetened shredded coconut

¼ cup vegan protein powder

¼ cup raw walnuts

½ cup chia seeds

¾ cup almond butter

¼ cup goji berries

2 pitted medjool dates

1 Tbsp maca powder

1 tsp cinnamon

1 tsp vanilla extract

1 tsp almond extract

Coating:

½ cup cocoa powder

¼ cup melted coconut oil

2 Tbsp maple syrup

Stevia to taste

Mix all ingredients, except coating ingredients, in a food processor bowl until blended thoroughly. Roll mixture into one inch balls. Place on cookie sheet and freeze for at least an hour.

In a small bowl, mix coating ingredients with a whisk. Spoon over each ball and place in freezer for 30 minutes until set.

SOUPS

Melon Soup

Serves 6

Melon Soup is a light and refreshing soup that is scintillating. It can be relished as a delightful breakfast on the hot days of summer. I love how bright and vibrant the orange color is, just like the sun. This is wonderful for breakfast, lunch or as a fresh and satisfying dessert.

3 cups fresh cantaloupe melon, chilled and peeled

1 ½ coconut water

½ cup fresh squeezed orange juice

1 tsp cinnamon

1 tsp lemon juice

3 dates, pitted and soaked for 2 hours

Pinch Cardamom, if desired

Cashew cream (see Extras)

Combine all ingredients, except cardamom and cashew cream, in a blender and blend until smooth. Serve warm or chill for 1 hour before serving. Serve with a pinch of cardamom and a drizzle of cashew cream.

Southwestern Pumpkin Chowder

Serves 6

This soup is rich and thick with southwestern flair. It is a favorite for those who love Mexican food but want something substantial but are watching their waistline. This chowder reminds me of enchilada soup, but better!

1 Tbsp extra virgin olive oil

4 cloves garlic, minced

2 tsp cumin

1 tsp chili powder - hot or mild

Pinch hot red pepper flakes (if desired)

1 – 15 oz. can pumpkin

1 – 15 oz. can fire roasted diced tomatoes with juice

1 – 8 oz. can green chilies, not drained

1 heaping cup roasted corn kernels

1 cup salsa

1 cup broth

1 cup water

2 cups coconut creamer

Sea salt and fresh ground pepper

Chopped cilantro, to taste - dried or fresh

Juice from 1 fresh lime

Heat the olive oil in a heavy soup pot and add the garlic, cumin, chili powder and pepper flakes; stir for one minute. Add the pumpkin, tomatoes, green chilies, corn, and salsa. Stir to combine. Add the broth and water. Bring to a gentle boil, then reduce heat to a simmer. While stirring, add the coconut creamer until desired consistency is attained. Season with sea salt and ground pepper to taste. Heat through gently over low heat. Serve topped with cilantro and lime juice.

Moroccan Chickpea Millet Soup

Serves 8

This soup is mildly sweet from the exotic spices and makes a tasty bowl during colder weather. I often eat this for breakfast in the winter when I want something warm and satisfying at the start of the day. It is delicious with a poached egg on top as the soft egg yolk offers a luxurious and velvety consistency.

2 Tbsp grape seed oil

1 medium onion, diced

2 cloves garlic, minced

1 cup celery, diced

1 cup sweet potato, peeled and diced

1 can cooked chickpeas

⅓ cup uncooked millet

1 ½ tsp ground cumin

¼ tsp turmeric

¼ tsp nutmeg

3 lemon slices

4 cups water

4 cups vegetable broth

1 tsp sea salt

Pinch of black pepper

Sauté onion, garlic, and celery in oil over medium heat for 5 minutes or until onion is soft. Add remaining ingredients and bring to a boil. Reduce heat and simmer for 20 minutes or until sweet potatoes and millet are cooked.

Clam Chowder

Serves 6

On our most recent trip to Cape Cod, I was fantasizing about the clam chowder I loved so much until I was diagnosed with food allergies. For the first time in many years, I felt underprivileged. I became determined to create my own version and although it is not pure white in color, I feel my version is a success.

4 slices peppered turkey bacon (optional)

2 Tbsp grape seed oil

1 cup onion, diced

1 cup celery, diced

½ cup carrot, finely diced

2 garlic cloves, minced

1 cup red potatoes, diced

16 oz. clam juice

1 bay leaf

2 - 6.5 oz. cans minced clams

2 cups coconut milk

½ cup sweet rice flour, tapioca flour, or potato starch

1 pint plain coconut creamer

Salt and black pepper to taste

Earth Balance soy free spread

Vegan cheddar style cheese, shredded

Finely chop bacon and cook in a cast iron pot with 2 Tbsp. grape seed oil. Remove and set aside when crispy.

In the same pot, sweat the onion, celery, carrot and garlic in the bacon fat for about a minute. Stir in potatoes and sauté another 5 minutes. Add clam juice and simmer until veggies are tender. Add clams with their juice and the coconut milk. In a small bowl, whisk the flour into the creamer and then add to soup. Simmer for 5 minutes. Season to taste.

Serve topped with bacon crumbles, a dollop of Earth Balance soy free spread and vegan cheese.

Mike's Vegetable Beef Soup

Serves 8

This recipe comes compliments of my husband, Mike. Although he doesn't have a vast repertoire of recipes, his recipe for vegetable beef soup is simple and delicious. You easily can make this a vegetarian soup by swapping out the beef stock for vegetable broth and using beans or chopped mushrooms instead of the beef. We also change this recipe based on what is in season, so it is not unusual to find our soup studded with beets, turnips or broccoli. This soup has the best flavor two days following preparation.

3 Tbsp grape seed oil, divided

2 ½ lbs. beef round roast

2 quarts water

4 carrots, diced

2 stalks celery, diced

1 garlic clove, minced

1 large onion, chopped

1 cup green beans, chopped

1 cup organic frozen corn kernels

1 cup frozen lima beans

1 cup frozen peas

2 large red skinned potatoes, chopped into 1" chunks

1 quart low sodium beef stock

1 large can no salt added tomato sauce

1 small can diced tomatoes

1 Tbsp gluten free Worcestershire sauce

1 Tbsp Italian herbs (basil, oregano, thyme, savory)

2 tsp sea salt

1 tsp black pepper

1 tsp celery seed

Chopped fresh parsley leaves

Heat 2 tablespoons of oil over high heat in a large stock pot. Add the roast and sear on each side. Next, pour in the water and bring to a boil. Reduce heat to a simmer, cover and allow beef to cook for 2 hours until tender. Remove the beef and set aside. Place the broth remaining in the fridge and allow to cool. Once the fat has solidified, pour the broth through a fine metal strainer and discard the fat, reserving the broth. Cut the beef into ½" pieces.

Using the same stock pot, sauté the carrots, celery, garlic, and onions in the remaining oil until soft. Add the green beans, corn, lima beans, corn and potatoes. Stir the reserved cooking broth, beef stock, tomato sauce and diced tomatoes. Bring to a boil. Add the beef back to pot and stir in Worcestershire sauce, Italian herbs, sea salt, pepper, and celery seed. Reduce heat to a simmer and cook for at least one hour.

Serve topped with fresh chopped parsley.

Chicken Noodle Soup

Serves 4

Perhaps the most difficult soup to give up when going gluten free is chicken noodle. Chicken noodle soup provides comfort and brings back fond memories of being a kid. Whether coming inside from playing in the snow or nursing a sickness, a piping hot bowl of protein-rich chicken soup will warm your body and soul.

2 Tbsp rice bran oil

1 cup carrots, diced

1 cup celery, diced

½ cup shallots, diced

6 cups chicken bone broth

2 cups cooked chicken, shredded

1 Tbsp dried thyme

2 tsp dried tarragon

Sea salt and pepper to taste

1 package thin vermicelli rice noodles, broken

In large pot, sauté veggies in oil until translucent, about 4 to 5 minutes. Pour in broth and bring to a boil. Reduce heat to a simmer and simmer 30 to 45 minutes. Add in cooked chicken and spices. Allow to heat through, about 10 minutes. Season to taste.

Meanwhile, cook rice noodles according to package directions. Drain, and rinse under cold water. Divide noodles among bowls and top with hot soup mixture. Store noodles separate from soup to retain their shape and resiliency.

Apricot Lentil Soup

Serves 4-6

All I can say about this recipe is yum! It is so hassle-free and easy to prepare and is a perfect recipe to start transitioning to a healthier lifestyle. Even the pickiest eaters and scrape to the bottom of their bowl of this thick, rich soup.

3 Tbsp extra virgin olive oil

1 large onion, chopped

2 cloves garlic, minced

2 medium carrots, finely diced

⅓ cup dried unsulphured apricots, chopped

1 ½ cups red lentils, rinsed

4 cups vegetable stock

1 large tomato, diced

½ tsp ground cumin

½ tsp dried thyme

½ tsp ground black pepper

Sea salt to taste

Sauté onion, garlic, carrots, and apricots in olive oil. Stir in lentils and stock and bring to a boil. Reduce heat and simmer 30 minutes. Add tomatoes, cumin, thyme, salt and pepper to taste, and simmer 10 minutes more. Puree ½ of the soup in a blender, then return to the pot and stir.

Vegetarian Split Pea Soup

Serves 4-6

I was never a fan of split pea soup until a friend and I prepared this meat-free version. I do not like ham and always found split pea soup to be too smoky for my taste. Instead, this soup uses plenty of fresh vegetables and coconut creamer that results in a thick and savory soup. If you wish a more smoky flavor, this is delicious topped with crispy pancetta. Delish!

1 lb. split peas, picked through and cooked according to package instructions

3 cups low sodium vegetable broth

1 cup plain coconut creamer

2 Tbsp extra virgin olive oil

3 celery stalks, diced

1 cup diced carrots

1 zucchini, diced

½ onion, diced

2 garlic cloves, minced

2 tsp dried thyme

2 bay leaves

1 tsp garlic powder

1 tsp onion powder

2 tsp sea salt

1 tsp black pepper

¼ tsp ground nutmeg

Parsley, garnish

Cook split peas according to package instructions.

In large pot, sauté veggies in olive oil until tender. Stir in spices and heat 1 minute. Add broth, peas and bring to a boil. Reduce heat and simmer 20-25 minutes. Remove bay leaves and puree with immersion blender. Stir in coconut creamer and heat through. Serve topped with fresh parsley.

Tomato Soup

Serves 6

Although tomato soup was never a favorite of mine growing up, it was for many people, especially my brother. I created this recipe with him in mind. Tom- this one's for you!

2 Tbsp extra virgin olive oil
1 onion, chopped
1 clove garlic, chopped
1 – 28 oz. can crushed tomatoes
2 cups low-sodium chicken broth
2 cups plain coconut creamer
Salt and pepper

Warm oil in a large saucepan over medium-high heat. Add onion and cook, stirring often, until softened. Add garlic and cook about 1 minute.

Add tomatoes and broth to saucepan, increase heat to high and bring to a boil. Stir or whisk constantly until slightly thickened, about 3 minutes. Stir in creamer.

Working in batches, carefully transfer soup to a blender and puree until smooth. Pour into a bowl until all soup is pureed. Season with salt and pepper.

Vegan Broccoli Cheese Soup

Serves 4

Who doesn't love cheesy soup? Enough said….

3 cups low sodium vegetable broth

1 cup water

1 pound broccoli crowns, trimmed and chopped (about 6 cups)

¼ cup onions, chopped finely

1 clove garlic, minced

1 14-oz. can cannellini beans, drained and rinsed

2 cups raw spinach

¼ tsp sea salt

¼ tsp ground white pepper

1 cup vegan cheese

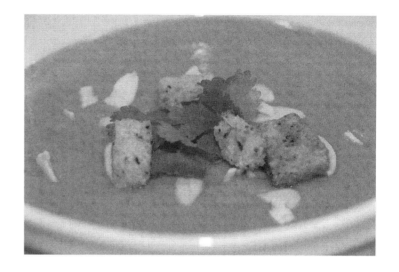

Bring broth and water to a boil in a medium saucepan over high heat. Add broccoli, onions and garlic; cover and cook until tender, about 8 minutes. Stir in beans, spinach, salt and pepper and cook until the beans are heated through, about 1 minute.

Place half the mixture into a blender with half the cheese. Puree until smooth and transfer to a bowl. Repeat with the remaining broccoli mixture and cheese. Serve hot.

Crock Pot White Turkey Chili

Makes 6-8 servings

There was a time when anything made with tomatoes made my joints ache, but I LOVE chili. I became determined to devise a recipe that would soothe my cravings for a spicy bowl of southwestern flavor without the residual pain that usually followed. This fits my needs perfectly.

2 lbs. ground turkey breast

1 ½ cups chicken or turkey stock

1 can cannellini beans, drained and rinsed

1 can chopped green chilies

1 onion, chopped

3 cloves garlic, minced

1 Tbsp ground cumin

1 Tbsp chili powder

1 tsp sea salt

½ tsp ground white pepper

2 Tbsp corn flour mixed with 1 Tbsp water

⅓ cup chopped fresh cilantro, garnish

½ fresh squeezed lime, garnish

In your slow cooker, add turkey, chicken stock, cooked or canned white kidney beans, chilies, onion, garlic, cumin, chili powder, salt and pepper. Stir. Cover and cook on high for 3 ½ hours, stirring several times. Add corn flour mixture about a half hour before serving and stir well. Serve topped with chopped cilantro and a squeeze of lime.

Veggie Chili

Serves 8

This dish pleases meat eaters and vegetarians alike due to the heartiness of the beans and warmth of the perfect blend of spices. Chili is perfect for the colder months and using fresh sweet potatoes during the fall harvest promises a satisfying and nutritious supper rich in beta carotene and immune boosting vitamin C.

1 Tbsp extra virgin olive oil

1 onion, diced

½ cup celery, chopped

1 cup sweet potato, diced

2 cups zucchini, diced

3 garlic cloves, minced

½ tsp sea salt

Black pepper to taste

1 Tbsp chili powder

2 tsp cumin

1 can kidney beans

2 ½ cups vegetable broth

1 cup water

28 oz. can crushed tomatoes

In a large pot over medium heat, add oil, onions, celery, sweet potatoes, zucchini, garlic, salt, pepper and spices, and stir thoroughly. Cover and allow to gently steam for 10 minutes, stirring occasionally.

Add the kidney beans to the pot with the vegetable broth, water, and crushed tomatoes and stir to combine. Decrease the heat to low, cover and simmer for approximately 45 minutes until the potatoes are tender. Serve warm.

Minestrone Soup

Serves 8

Minestrone soup was a big part of my childhood as we ate A LOT of soup. This was one of my favorites because I loved the variety of vegetables, Italian flavors and fullness it provided. Traditionally, minestrone contains pasta, but I find that using just beans alone still make for a satisfying and flavorful bowl of steamy perfection.

2 Tbsp extra virgin olive oil

1 small head fennel, diced

1 onion, diced

2 large cloves garlic, minced

3 carrots, peeled and diced

3 stalks celery, diced

1 yellow summer squash, diced

1 zucchini, diced

1 can diced tomatoes, drained

1 Tbsp dried oregano

1 Tbsp dried basil

1 tsp sea salt

2 quarts vegetable stock

1 can kidney beans

Add olive oil to large pot and sauté fennel, onion, garlic, carrots and celery for a few minutes. Add squash and zucchini and cook for 3 to 4 minutes longer. Stir in tomatoes, seasonings and stock and bring to a boil. Add beans and reduce heat. Simmer for 60 minutes.

Creamy Celeriac Soup

Serves 6

My husband adores celery and I love celery root. This soup is luscious and is a great way to use up your cellar vegetables. It is sweet and rich and can be modified by using with other root vegetables such as kohlrabi, rutabaga or sweet potatoes. Enjoy!

2 Tbsp extra virgin olive oil

½ cup onion, diced

1 large celery root, peeled and cut into 1" chunks

1 cup Yukon gold potatoes, diced

1 can cannellini beans with liquid

4 cups vegetable stock

1 large apple, peeled and diced

1 cup coconut creamer

Pinch allspice

Sea salt and black pepper to taste

¼ cup green onions, sliced

Heat oil in large pot over medium heat. Add onion and cook until onions are soft. Add celery root, potato, beans and vegetable stock. Reduce heat and simmer about 20 minutes.

Add the apple, coconut creamer and allspice and cook for 5 minutes. Remove saucepan from heat and puree using an immersion blender and season with salt and pepper. Serve topped with green onions.

Creamy Roasted Red Pepper, Tomato and Artichoke Soup

Serves 6

I love making soups, especially when it is so easy to prepare a piping bowl of heart-warming nourishment in minutes. This soup is extremely inexpensive and tastes much better than the store bought varieties. I guarantee that you will find it difficult to settle for canned soup after tasting this delectable homemade version.

1 entire head of garlic

2 Tbsp extra virgin olive oil

1 onion, diced

1 large can crushed San Marzano tomatoes

1 red pepper, roasted, or 1 large jar roasted red peppers, drained

2 large jars marinated artichoke hearts, drained

2 cups vegetable stock, heated on stove

1 Tbsp ground fennel seed

2 tsp dried thyme

1 cup plain coconut creamer

Sea salt and pepper to taste

Preheat oven to 350° F. Cut off and discard the top ¼ of the garlic bulb and wrap the rest of the bulb in aluminum foil. Bake the garlic for 45 to 60 minutes. Remove and allow to cool. Squeeze the garlic bulb until all of the roasted garlic paste is removed. Set aside.

To prepare the soup, heat the oil in large pot and sauté onions until soft. Stir in the tomatoes, peppers, artichokes and roasted garlic paste and bring to a boil. Remove from heat and blend with an immersion blender until desired consistency. Pour the soup back into the pot and add the stock, fennel, thyme, and creamer and heat through. Season with salt and pepper.

SALADS

Happy Hempseed Salad

Serves 2

What a wonderful way to pack some protein and omega-3 fatty acids into a crunchy salad with a piquant dressing. For me, it is paradise when paired with a bowl of steamy soup.

4 cups baby spinach

½ cup hemp seeds

2 scallions, sliced

2 celery ribs, finely chopped

4 carrots, shaved

1 medium cucumber, finely chopped

¼ cup sunflower seeds

¼ cup dried unsweetened cherries, soaked for 1 hour

1 Tbsp fresh basil, chiffonade

1 Tbsp fresh mint, chopped

Combine all ingredients in a bowl. Toss with dressing.

<u>Dressing:</u>

2 Tbsp lime juice

2 Tbsp walnut oil

1 Tbsp apple cider vinegar

1 Tbsp raw honey

Pinch sea salt

Whisk dressing ingredients together. Pour over salad ingredients and toss to coat.

Fall Fruit Salad with Maple Vinaigrette

Serves 2

Can you tell that autumn is my favorite season, especially when it comes to the bounty of fall flavors? I eat salads year-round, so in order for them to be satisfying during cooler temperatures, I use seasonal fruits and vegetables to ensure maximum taste, texture and nutrition.

4 cups salad mix of your choice

4 celery stalks, thinly sliced

1 plum, halved, cored, and thinly sliced

1 apple, halved, cored, and thinly sliced

1 pear, halved, cored, and thinly sliced

⅓ cup pomegranate seeds

⅓ cup sunflower seeds

In a large bowl, combine salad mix, celery, plum, apple, pear, and pomegranate seeds. Toss with dressing. Serve salad sprinkled with sunflower seeds.

Vinaigrette:

2 Tbsp extra virgin olive oil

1 Tbsp cider vinegar

2 tsp maple syrup

1 ½ Tbsp Dijon mustard

Pinch cinnamon

Pinch ground ginger

Coarse sea salt and ground pepper to taste

Whisk together olive oil, cider vinegar, maple syrup, and Dijon mustard. Season dressing with cinnamon, ginger, sea salt and pepper to taste.

Cauliflower Salad

Serves 8

This salad is a home cook's favorite because it is a raw salad prepared the day before serving. It involves little chopping and is compiled quickly. The flavors penetrate into the vegetables overnight and make them crisp yet tender. Kids love this salad and it is a great way to introduce them to new vegetables.

1 medium head cauliflower

1 head organic iceberg lettuce, shredded

½ cup coconut bacon (see Extras)

1 cup frozen green peas, thawed

2 large carrots, diced small

¼ cup red onion, finely chopped

½ cup vegan mayonnaise

½ cup unsweetened plain coconut milk yogurt

1 Tbsp Dijon mustard

2 Tbsp raw honey

¼ cup nutritional yeast

Add cauliflower to food processor and pulse until chopped into small pieces. Pour into large bowl. Add iceberg lettuce to bowl with cauliflower. Add the coconut bacon, peas, carrots, and onion and toss to combine.

In a small bowl, stir together the mayonnaise, yogurt, mustard, honey and yeast. Stir the mayonnaise mixture into the vegetable blend to coat. Refrigerate overnight. Serve cold.

Dijon Carrot Apple Salad

Serves 4

Salads are not always a bowl of lettuce, which isn't always satisfying, particularly in winter months. The zing of this salad is delightful and gets better the longer it sits. Enjoy!

1 cup shredded carrots

1 small apple, diced

2 stalks celery, diced

¼ cup chopped kale

½ cup fresh pomegranate seeds

¼ cup raw pumpkin seeds

2 Tbsp Dijon mustard

2 Tbsp extra virgin olive oil

2 Tbsp lemon juice

2 tsp raw honey

1 clove garlic, minced

1 Tbsp apple cider vinegar

½ tsp sea salt

¼ tsp ground black pepper

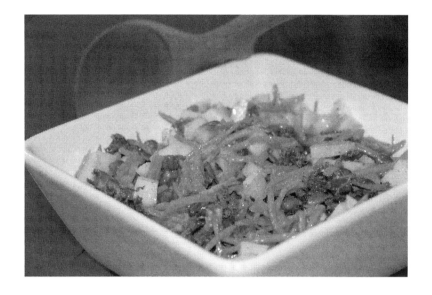

Combine carrots, apple, celery, kale, pomegranate, and pumpkin seeds in a large bowl. In a small bowl, whisk remaining ingredients. Pour over carrot mixture and toss to coat, seasoning to taste.

Super Green Chopped Salad

Serves 4

Although many restaurants offer chopped salads, you likely haven't had one quite like this. I tend to be reckless in the kitchen, pairing unusual ingredients together and rolling the dice. In this circumstance, I created a masterpiece of flavor that is not only healthy and delicious, but pleasing to the eye as well. I could eat this anytime, even for dessert.

1 avocado

2 Tbsp red wine vinegar

1 Tbsp extra virgin olive oil

1 Tbsp lemon juice

1 Tbsp raw honey

1 tsp Dijon mustard

4 cups raw kale, chopped

2 cup shredded Brussels sprouts

1 cup broccoli slaw

4 green onions, chopped

1 small cucumber, seeded and diced

1 cup chopped apple

2 Tbsp unsweetened coconut flakes

2 Tbsp pumpkin seeds

3 Tbsp dried fruit of choice

Pinch sea salt and pepper

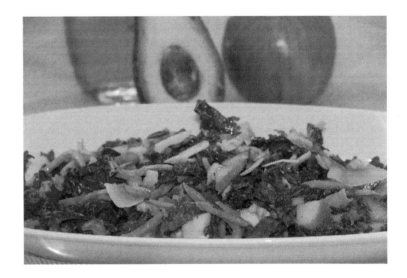

Place the avocado, vinegar, olive oil, lemon juice, honey, and mustard in a large bowl. Add the raw kale, Brussels sprouts and broccoli slaw and using your hands, massage the wet ingredients into the vegetables until the kale becomes soft and wilted. Stir in the green onions, cucumber, apple, coconut flakes, pumpkin seeds, and dried fruit until evenly distributed. Season to taste with salt and pepper and serve.

Winter Squash Salad with Dragonfruit Dressing

Serves 2

This is a perfect dish to use up the overwhelming bounty of squash after the summer harvest. It is a stunning autumn dish with eye-popping, bright orange squash chunks, crisp green spinach and pink dressing. The tanginess of the dragon fruit is unusual and yet what I love most about this dressing.

2 cups diced and roasted butternut squash

2 cups baby spinach

½ cup pomegranate seeds

½ cup sautéed chopped onions

1 apple, diced

¼ cup walnuts

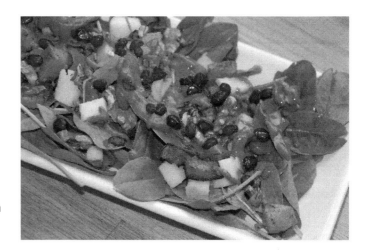

Prepare all the vegetables and place them in a salad bowl.

Dragon Fruit Tahini Dressing:

2 Tbsp coconut vinegar

2 Tbsp dried dragon fruit, chopped

Zest of a lemon

Juice of a lemon

1 Tbsp tahini

1 Tbsp purified water

1 Tbsp raw honey

¼ tsp sea salt

White pepper to taste

Blend together the dressing ingredients until smooth and set aside. Serve salad drizzled with dressing.

Celery and Broccoli Salad

Serves 4

This salad is spectacular with the various shades of green and red specks from the onion. It is crunchy, slightly sweet and even more delightful after sitting in the fridge for a day or two.

1 head broccoli, cut into florets

2 zucchini squash, trimmed and cut into fine julienne (matchstick) strips

2 celery stalks, chopped

1 small bunch radishes, trimmed sliced

1 cup snap peas, chopped

¼ cup red onion, chopped

¼ cup pumpkin seeds

Dressing:

1 Tbsp Dijon mustard

2 Tbsp coconut aminos

1 tsp toasted sesame oil

3 Tbsp apple juice

Sea salt and pepper to taste

Bring a medium saucepan of water to a boil. Add the broccoli and blanch for 2 to 3 minutes. Strain and run under the cold water tap until completely cold.

Place the broccoli in a large bowl with the remaining vegetables. In a small bowl, whisk together the dressing ingredients and pour over the salad. Toss to coat and serve.

Sweet & Savory Quinoa Salad

Serves 2-3

Quinoa is a wonderful grain-like seed that provides iron, protein, B vitamins and many other nutrients. I love the texture and earthiness of quinoa, especially since rice can be boring and unappetizing at times. Quinoa is flavorful and astonishing when cooked in green tea or broth. I recommend sampling all colors of quinoa to find your favorite variety.

1 cup quinoa

2 cups low-sodium vegetable broth

2 large carrots, peeled and diced

3 large celery stalks, peeled and diced

1 large red bell pepper, seeded and diced

3 scallions, sliced

¼ cup dried cherries

¼ cup chopped pecans

Dressing:

3 Tbsp minced parsley

½ cup rice vinegar

2 Tbsp coconut water

1 Tbsp maple syrup

1 Tbsp grape seed oil

2 garlic cloves, chopped fine

Pinch sea salt

Rinse the quinoa in a fine-mesh sieve under running water for 1 minute. Bring the broth to a boil in a medium saucepan. Slowly add the quinoa and bring to a boil. Lower the heat, cover, and simmer for 15 minutes. Refrigerate until cool.

Meanwhile, prepare place the carrots, celery, pepper, scallions, cherries, and pecans in a salad bowl. Add quinoa to the vegetables. In a separate bowl, whisk together the dressing ingredients. Toss with quinoa and veggies until coated well. Refrigerate leftovers within 2-3 hours.

Anti-Aging Salad

Serves 2

The Anti-Aging Salad is one of my go-to lunches when I have leftover quinoa in the fridge. It provides hydration, can provide hormone balance, and is full of antioxidants. It has a pepper taste from the arugula that is subtle yet enjoyable. This salad is definitely a crowd pleaser.

4 cups baby arugula

½ cup roasted watermelon seeds

1 cup mixed berries

1 small watermelon radish, thinly sliced

½ cup cooked quinoa

1 avocado, diced

Combine all ingredients in large bowl. Toss with dressing.

Dressing:

2 Tbsp champagne vinegar

½ tsp matcha powder

2 Tbsp avocado oil

½ Tbsp raw honey

1 tsp Dijon mustard

Salt and white pepper to taste

Whisk all dressing ingredients in bowl until slightly frothy.

Fall Bean and Squash Salad

Serves 8-10

Bean salad is a fantastic way to introduce beans to people because it allows them to try multiple beans at once. Each bean has its own distinct taste and texture, and when paired with crisp vegetables and the acidity of the dressing, the flavor pops. The vibrant autumn colors speckled throughout make this dish hard to resist.

2 Tbsp extra virgin olive oil

1 Tbsp fresh lemon juice

1 Tbsp coconut nectar

½ tsp coarse sea salt

Freshly ground pepper, to taste

1 can chickpeas, drained and rinsed

1 can red kidney beans, drained and rinsed

1 cup roasted butternut squash

½ cup frozen lima beans, thawed

1 small zucchini, diced into ½" squares

1 small yellow squash, diced into ½" squares

¼ cup red onion, diced

½ cup red bell pepper, finely diced

1 Tbsp chopped fresh basil

In a small bowl, whisk together olive oil, lemon juice, coconut nectar, sea salt and pepper. Set aside. In a large bowl, combine remaining ingredients. Pour the olive oil mixture into the vegetable mixture and toss to combine. Chill for one hour before serving.

Note: For a summer bean salad, substitute the butternut squash for ½ cup fresh corn kernels and ½ cup diced cherry tomatoes. I also substitute the lemon juice with lime juice.

Grapefruit Jicama Salad

Serves 4

Light, cleansing, refreshing and crisp. If you find grapefruit too sour for you, try using a mandarin orange or clementine segments in exchange to produce an equally cooling salad for those hot summer days.

2 ruby red grapefruit, extra juice reserved

2 cups shredded endive

1 small bulb of fennel, cored and thinly sliced

1 jicama, peeled and cut into sticks

2 avocados, peeled, pitted and cut into chunks

½ cup fresh raspberries

2 Tbsp extra virgin olive oil

2 Tbsp coconut water

1 Tbsp apple cider vinegar

1 packet stevia

1 tsp Dijon mustard

¼ tsp sea salt

Pinch of freshly ground pepper

1 Tbsp chopped fennel fronds

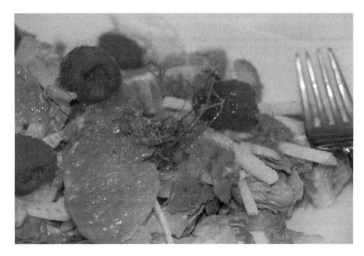

Cut the grapefruit into segments and set aside in a medium bowl, retaining the remaining grapefruit. Add shredded endive, fennel, jicama, avocados and raspberries and set aside.

In a small bowl, squeeze any remaining grapefruit juice from the fruit. Add the olive oil, coconut water, vinegar, stevia, mustard, salt and pepper to the grapefruit juice and whisk until smooth. Stir in the fennel fronds. Pour over salad and toss to combine.

Curried Carrot & Zucchini Salad

Serves 4

I appreciate carrots because they are sweet, crunchy and very portable. I concocted this recipe after I had the pleasure of enjoying a similar salad at a potluck party years ago. This lip-smacking salad uses a twist of citrus and is best chilled overnight so the flavors fully infuse into the carrot and zucchini shreds.

1 lb. carrots, peeled and shredded

2 large zucchini, shredded and strained

¼ cup golden raisins

¼ cup crushed pineapple

¼ cup vegan mayonnaise

2 Tbsp chopped walnuts

2 scallions, sliced

1 tsp curry powder

Juice and zest of an orange

Salt and pepper to taste

Combine all ingredients in bowl and toss until well combined.

Refreshing Citrus and Root Veggie Salad

Serves 2

This garden-fresh salad is healthy and elegant. It keeps well in the fridge for days (keep the avocado and arugula out for best results). The flavors meld together perfectly and is robust with antioxidants and fiber. It is fantastic for breakfast with a slice of gluten free toast topped with mashed avocado and alfalfa sprouts on hot summer days.

1 jicama, chopped finely

1 fennel bulb, sliced thinly on a mandolin

½ cup sliced radishes

2 limes, peeled and segmented (marinated in water and stevia for at least an hour)

2 Tbsp fresh cilantro, chopped

¼ cup pomegranate seeds

¼ cup chopped macadamia nuts

1 avocado, pitted and diced

8 large romaine lettuce leaves

Dressing:

2 Tbsp lime juice

2 Tbsp avocado oil

1 Tbsp coconut vinegar

1 Tbsp raw honey or to taste

1 small clove garlic, minced

Sea salt and pepper to taste

In a small bowl, whisk together oil, lime juice, vinegar, honey, and garlic. Set aside.

In a medium bowl, combine jicama, fennel, radishes, limes, and cilantro. Pour the dressing over the jicama and fennel mixture and toss to coat. Add in pomegranate, nuts, and avocado and toss again. Season with salt and pepper to taste. Serve atop lettuce leaves.

Unruly Caesar Salad

Serves 2

This salad is not traditional, but it is certainly a tasty alternative to the restaurant favorite.

1 large head romaine lettuce, chopped

½ cup chickpeas, drained and rinsed

2 Tbsp pepitas

1 brown rice tortilla, toasted and chopped into small pieces

Serve tossed with Caesar dressing. (See dressing recipes in Extras)

Tropical Cabbage Salad

Serves 6

Cabbage is a wonderful vegetable for cleansing and detox. It is low in calories and is acts as a sponge when marinated or served with a sauce. This coleslaw spin-off is free of eggs and saturated fats and has a subtle tropical sweetness from the mango and coconut shreds. Perfect for any season!

¼ cup coconut vinegar

¼ cup vegan mayonnaise

½ medium avocado

2 Tbsp pineapple juice

2 Tbsp coconut water

1 Tbsp coconut nectar

1 Tbsp shredded coconut

1 tsp fresh ginger, grated

½ tsp sea salt plus extra if needed

White pepper to taste

1 small head green cabbage, shredded

¼ cup chopped red onion

1 large mango, diced

⅓ cup macadamia nuts, chopped

To prepare the dressing, in a blender, blend the vinegar, mayonnaise, avocado, pineapple juice, coconut water, coconut nectar, coconut shreds, and grated ginger.

Toss the cabbage, red onion, mango, and macadamia nuts with the dressing and an extra pinch of salt. Let the salad sit for 5 minutes; taste again and adjust the seasoning as needed. Chill for one hour before serving.

SIDES

Oven Roasted Vegetables

Serves 6

The easiest way to increase your vegetable intake is to try making different vegetables using a variety of methods, such as roasting, braising, steaming, sautéing or by consuming raw. This recipe is also helpful when trying new vegetables because you can pair them with your favorites without dominating the dish with the flavor of the newly introduced vegetable.

5 whole garlic cloves

1 cup acorn or butternut squash, diced

1 medium sweet potato, diced

1 cup turnips or rutabaga, diced

½ cup parsnips or carrots, diced

1 large onion, cut into sliced

1 zucchini, sliced or diced

1 large beet, diced

2 Tbsp extra virgin olive oil

2 Tbsp balsamic vinegar

1 tsp salt

½ tsp black pepper

1 cup broccoli, chopped

Preheat oven to 425°F.

Place the garlic and all vegetables, except broccoli, on a large cookie sheet with edges. Drizzle with the olive oil, balsamic vinegar, sea salt and pepper and toss to coat. Roast the vegetables for 20 minutes and add broccoli. Stir in the broccoli and continue to bake for an additional 20 minutes or until soft and slightly browned along edges.

Easy Roasted Vegetable Soup

Serves 4

2 cups roasted vegetables

2 cups chicken or vegetable stock

Salt and pepper to taste

Combine all ingredients in blender. Blend until smooth. Heat and serve.

Dijon Roasted Brussels Sprouts

Serves 6

Even those who despise Brussels sprouts find this dish impossible to hate. The Dijon mustard paired with honey imparts a caramel-like flavor that makes the taste buds sing.

¼ cup extra virgin olive oil

2 Tbsp Dijon mustard

2 Tbsp honey

1 Tbsp gluten free tamari

2 tsp dried tarragon

1 Tbsp Earth Balance soy free spread

2 lbs. Brussels sprouts, cored and quartered

Whisk the first six ingredients together in medium size bowl. Toss in Brussels sprouts to coat evenly. Spread the sprouts in a single layer on a baking sheet, rotating and stirring the sprouts after 15 minutes. Return to oven and roast an additional 10 to --15 minutes.

Quinoa Stuffing

Serves 4

It seems that no holiday is complete without a bowl of stuffing. Many gluten free stuffing blends available in the stores are extremely high in sodium, have little flavor and are difficult to find. Look no further! Your guests will be wowed by this side dish. And, the leftovers are fantastic with roasted or fresh vegetables such as onions, carrots, beets or winter squash. If you are a gravy lover, a chickpea or mushroom gravy adds velvety richness.

2 Tbsp extra virgin olive oil

⅓ cup sliced leeks, white and light green parts only

2 cups cooked quinoa

½ tsp sea salt

¼ cup chopped cashews

¼ cup chopped unsulphured dried apricots

½ cup shredded kale

1 Tbsp maple syrup

1 Tbsp coconut aminos

1 tsp lemon zest

2 tsp dried thyme

½ tsp dried sage

Heat olive oil in large skillet over medium heat. Sauté leeks until softened and pour into a bowl. Add remaining ingredients and season to taste with salt and pepper. Serve warm or at room temperature.

Italian Rice Bites

Makes 10 servings

Rice Bites are my favorite single serving side dishes. Adults and kids alike savor these Italian crispy morsels because they are versatile, easy to make and make wonderful leftovers. The trick is baking them long enough to have a crispy exterior and a warm, gooey inside. I highly suggest using home-made pasta sauce for dipping as jarred sauces often are too sweet or salty.

2 cups cooked brown rice

Powdered egg replacer for 1 egg

3 Tbsp ground flax mixed with

1 Tbsp warm water

1 small onion, diced

4 cloves of garlic, minced

½ cup fresh basil, chiffonade

⅓ cup diced tomatoes

⅓ diced artichokes

½ cup vegan shredded mozzarella cheese

1 tsp ground fennel

½ tsp sea salt

2 Tbsp extra virgin olive oil

¼ cup nutritional yeast

Pasta sauce, for dipping

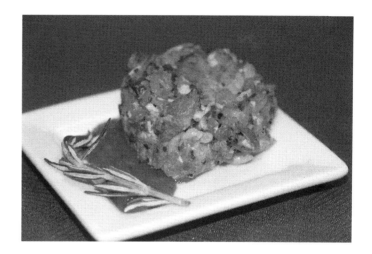

Preheat oven to 425°F.

In a large bowl, combine cooked rice with remaining ingredients, except pasta sauce; mix well to combine. Scoop into greased muffin tins and press down with back of spoon. Bake for 25 minutes or until golden brown and crispy. Remove from oven; set aside to cool for 10 minutes. Serve with pasta sauce for dipping.

Southwestern Sweet Bake

Serves 4

I find the traditional sweet potato dishes that incorporate sugary ingredients like maple syrup, cranberries and apples too overpowering. I do, however, relish the combination of sweet potatoes with spicy seasonings. It is pleasing to the palate and allows you to eat your garden's abundance creatively. Be sure to incorporate this spicy dish in your meal rotation schedule.

2 Tbsp extra virgin olive oil

¼ cup water

2 cups peeled sweet potato, sliced

½ cup sliced onion

½ red pepper, diced

1 jalapeno, diced finely

½ cup sliced shiitake mushrooms

2 cloves garlic, minced

½ cup unsweetened plain coconut milk yogurt

½ cup shredded vegan cheese

½ cup cashew cream (from extras section)

1 Tbsp ground cumin

1 tsp chili powder

1 tsp sea salt

1 avocado, diced

½ cup fresh cilantro leaves, chopped

½ cup salsa

10 organic corn tortilla chips, crushed

Heat oil and water in a medium sauté pan over medium high heat. Add sweet potato, onions, red bell pepper and jalapeno and cook until sweet potatoes soften a bit, stirring occasionally for 5 to 7 minutes. Stir in mushrooms and garlic and cook for 2 more minutes. Stir in yogurt, cheese, cashew cream, cumin, chili powder and salt. Pour into casserole dish and bake at 400°F until bubbly, about 10 minutes. Top with diced avocado, cilantro, salsa, and tortilla chips.

Rice Pilaf

Serves 5

My belief is that rice pilaf is underrated. If prepared well, it offers tender grains accented with savory and sweet flavors. This side dish is earthy, has a nutty nuance and offers a perfect balance of flavor.

3 Tbsp Earth Balance soy free spread
1 shallot, thinly sliced
¼ cup finely chopped carrot
1 ½ tsp sea salt
½ tsp ground black pepper
1 ½ cups basmati brown rice
½ cup wild rice
1 ½ cups vegetable broth
1 ½ cups water
1 bay leaf
1 sprig fresh rosemary
½ cup dried cranberries
2 Tbsp maple syrup

Melt the Earth Balance with the shallot and carrots in a medium saucepan over medium heat. Season with salt and pepper and cook until the shallots and carrots are soft. Add the brown and wild rice and stir until coated with the Earth Balance. Increase the heat to medium-high and allow the rice to toast for about 3 to 4 minutes, stirring occasionally.

Stir in the broth, water, bay leaf, and rosemary. Bring to a simmer over low heat, cover, and cook until all the broth has been absorbed by the rice and the rice is tender, about 20 to 25 minutes. Remove from the heat and let set for 5 minutes. Discard the rosemary and bay leaf. Fluff the rice with a fork, add cranberries and maple syrup and serve.

Warm German Potato Salad

Serves 6

German Potato salad served warm is rich, tangy and offers a unique dimension of flavor. The vinegar and mustard soak into the potato and render a perfect balance of sweet and sour. I add green beans and diced pimento pepper to the mix for protein, extra nutrients and color.

1 lb. baby red potatoes, cut into chunks

½ lb. green beans, cut into 2-inch pieces

2 Tbsp white balsamic vinegar

¼ cup vegan mayonnaise

2 Tbsp grainy mustard

¼ cup chopped fresh parsley

2 Tbsp chopped fresh dill

2 Tbsp chopped pimento peppers

½ tsp sea salt

¼ tsp black pepper

6 small scallions, chopped

Cook potatoes in pot of boiling salted water 8 minutes, or until tender. Add green beans during last minute of cooking. Drain potatoes and green beans and place in a large bowl.

In a small bowl, combine vinegar, mayonnaise, mustard, parsley, dill, pimento peppers, sea salt and black pepper. Stir until well combined. Pour over potatoes and beans, add scallions, and toss to coat.

Roasted Cauliflower with Apple and Dill

Serves 4

I certainly did not like cauliflower much until I began to experiment with it. Roasting cauliflower brings out a slightly nutty taste and results in a tender yet slightly crispy texture. This side dish can be made into a simple entrée by placing on a bed of fresh spinach and shredded carrot with a light splash of champagne vinaigrette and chopped macadamia nuts.

1 cauliflower, about 1 ½ pounds, core removed and separated into florets

½ large onion, cut into ¼ inch thick slices from root to tip

1 large unpeeled apple, cored and coarsely diced

3 Tbsp extra virgin olive oil

¾ tsp sea salt

3 Tbsp dried cranberries

¼ cup plus 2 Tbsp coarsely chopped dill weed

Preheat oven to 425°F.

Toss together the cauliflower, onion, apple, olive oil, and sea salt in a large shallow baking dish and spread the ingredients out into a single layer. Bake for 20 to 30 minutes, stirring once or twice along the way, until some of the edges of the cauliflower begin to brown. Stir in the cranberries and continue to bake about 10 more minutes, stirring another time or two, or until most of the edges of the cauliflower are browned. Sprinkle with the dill, stir again, and scoop into a serving dish.

Slow Cooker Vegetarian Baked Beans

Serves 12

I lived on baked beans in college. I remember when I was small and my mother would make a batch in a bean crock on the weekends. Beans are a cost effective and extraordinary source of vegetarian protein. Meat eaters can add some pork, ham or bacon, but I prefer the vegetarian version. Soaking the beans for several days helps remove the indigestible starch and helps activate the enzymes necessary for proper breakdown and assimilation of the nutrients.

3 cups dried navy beans

3 cups vegetable broth

1 - 6 oz. can tomato paste

1 Tbsp Worcestershire sauce

¼ cup brown sugar

2 Tbsp maple syrup

2 Tbsp molasses (not blackstrap)

2 Tbsp dried mustard

2 garlic cloves, minced

¼ cup sautéed chopped onion

2 tsp sea salt

¼ tsp black pepper

Soak the beans 5 days before making beans, making certain to drain, rinse and refill the beans twice each day.

Drain beans and rinse off. Put beans into slow cooker. Add all the remaining ingredients and stir. Cover and cook for 12 hours on low.

Creamy Macaroni and Cheese

Serves 8

This spin on macaroni and cheese uses winter squash. The orange color is familiar to kids and is a much healthier approach to the family favorite. It is certain to win over those used to orange rubber hoses, as my mother called them. It combines creamy cashew, sweet squash and salty miso to mimic the macaroni and cheese we all grew up on.

1 – 16oz. package cooked gluten free pasta

2 cups non-dairy milk (soy, rice, almond, hazelnut, hemp, oat —your choice)

6 Tbsp cornstarch or arrowroot

¼ cup Earth Balance soy free spread

1 ¼ cup raw cashews

1 butternut squash, steamed

¼ cup chopped onion, sweated

1 cup vegan mozzarella

½ cup nutritional yeast

2 Tbsp miso paste

2 tsp onion powder

1 tsp sea salt

1 tsp garlic powder

½ tsp paprika

½ tsp turmeric

¼ tsp ground white pepper

Preheat oven to 425°F.

Combine the milk, cornstarch and Earth Balance in a saucepan and bring to a gentle boil. Decrease the heat to low-medium, cover and simmer, stirring occasionally for 10 minutes or until the thickener is dissolved.

Add the cashews, squash, onion, vegan cheese, nutritional yeast, miso, and spices to a high speed blender. With the blender running, pour in the milk mixture and run until smooth and creamy. Combine the cheese mixture with cooked pasta and pour into baking dish. Bake for or 20 to 30 minutes, until golden and bubbly.

Jicama and Veggie Salad

Serves 6

This is a delectable and creamy salad similar to potato salad but free of white starches. This recipe is ideal for those who are seeking a diabetic-friendly treat. Of course you can always substitute potatoes, if you desire the traditional version. I adore jicama so I strive to use it as it often results in spectacular dishes.

Salad Ingredients:

1 lb. jicama, peeled and cubed

1 cup green beans, chopped

1 shallot, thinly sliced

¼ cup finely diced red onion

½ tsp sea salt

1 cup corn

1 large seedless cucumber, diced

1 roasted red bell pepper, diced

1 avocado, diced

½ cup sliced almonds

1 cup kidney beans, drained and rinsed

Dressing:

6 oz. plain unsweetened coconut milk yogurt

¼ cup vegan mayonnaise

2 Tbsp coconut or apple cider vinegar

1 clove garlic, minced

¼ cup extra virgin olive oil

Salt and freshly ground pepper, to taste

2-3 Tbsp fresh dill, chopped

¼ cup fresh parsley, chopped

Combine all salad ingredients in a large bowl. Top with dressing (whisk all ingredients together). Toss to coat. This salad is best when chilled overnight.

Broccoli Cheese Casserole

Serves 6

This recipe was adapted from my grandmother's recipe. I removed the highly processed "cheese food" and made a dairy free version that is just as delicious as the original. People who don't care for broccoli even beg me to make it for them.

2 - 10 oz. packages frozen chopped broccoli

1 small onion, diced

4 Tbsp Earth Balance soy free spread

2 Tbsp sweet rice flour

½ cup water or coconut milk

1 cup "cheese" (below)

3 beaten eggs

½ cup crushed gluten free crackers or bread crumbs

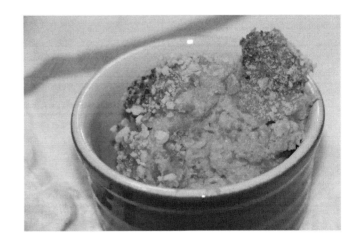

Preheat oven to 325°F.

Cook broccoli according to package instructions. Meanwhile, sauté onions in Earth Balance until soft. Whisk in sweet rice flour. Add water. Cook over low heat, until thick and mixture comes to a boil. Stir in "cheese". Add beaten eggs. Drain broccoli well and stir into sauce and eggs until blended. Pour into greased baking dish and cover with crumbs. Bake for 40 to 45 minutes.

"Cheese"

1 cup raw cashews

3 Tbsp lemon juice

1 tsp onion juice

¼ tsp garlic powder

2 ½ cups filtered water

4 oz. pimentos, drained

2 Tbsp nutritional yeast

1 tsp sea salt

Place all ingredients in a high speed blender and blend until thick and smooth.

Italian Bean & Broccoli Sauté

Serves 4

If I am presented with an amazing array of desserts or a bowl of beans and veggies, I always will opt for the vegetables. Call me crazy, but vegetables seem to warm my heart and soul. I find vegetables to be very grounding for me and incorporating vegetarian dishes into my meal rotation is very important to me. I added the broccoli for a spin on the traditional Minestra (Greens n' Beans) dish found in many Italian restaurants.

2 Tbsp extra virgin olive oil, plus more for drizzling

1 small red onion, sliced

3 cloves garlic, crushed

2 Tbsp tomato paste

2 cups broccoli

1 cup vegetable stock

2 cups kale, roughly chopped

2 cups spinach, roughly chopped

½ cup fresh cherry or grape tomatoes

1 – 15 oz. can cannellini beans

1 Tbsp fresh thyme

1 Tbsp fresh oregano

¼ cup fresh basil

½ teaspoon salt

Pepper to taste

Heat olive oil in a sauté pan, and then add onions, garlic and tomato paste. Sauté until onions begin to soften. Add broccoli and stock, cover pan, and steam until broccoli is tender and water is gone. Add kale, spinach and tomatoes and sauté one minute. Add beans and fresh herbs and continue to simmer until flavors meld together and beans are warm. Add salt and pepper to taste. Garnish with extra virgin olive oil and enjoy.

Roasted Roots & Fruits with Creamy Balsamic Drizzle

Serves 6

Roasted vegetables are a mainstay in my household and I eat them several times a week. The balsamic vinegar in this dish is remarkable as it adds zing character to this dish. In addition, the verdant balsamic blend gives the veggies character, which makes it easier to get kids to clean their plates.

1 red onion, sliced thinly

1 parsnip, peeled and diced

1 zucchini, sliced

1 rutabaga, peeled and diced

1 celery root, peeled and diced

6 Tbsp extra virgin olive oil, divided

1 cup grapes, halved

2 small pears, quartered

¼ cup walnut halves

1 avocado

¼ cup extra virgin olive oil

¼ cup balsamic vinegar

1 Tbsp Dijon mustard

2 tsp dried thyme

1 clove garlic

1 shallot, minced

1 tsp sea salt

½ tsp black pepper

Preheat oven to 425°F.

Place the onion, parsnip, zucchini, rutabaga, and celery root on baking sheet. Drizzle with 3 tablespoons of olive oil and place in oven. Bake for 25 minutes, remove and add the grapes and pears. Bake for an additional 15 minutes. Remove from oven, sprinkle with walnuts and set aside.

In a blender, blend the avocado, 3 tablespoons of olive oil, balsamic vinegar, mustard, thyme, garlic, shallot, sea salt and pepper on high speed until creamy and thick. Drizzle over veggies.

Corn Pudding

Serves 8

If you are seeking a warm and heart-healthy alternative to the traditional corn pudding found on the holiday table, look no further! This corn pudding rises nicely and has a buttery-smooth texture mixed with tender bits of corn. A real favorite among kids!

Cooking spray

2 Tbsp Earth Balance soy free spread, melted

1 – 16 oz. package frozen corn, thawed

1 ¾ cups boxed coconut milk

1 ½ cups fine organic yellow cornmeal

½ cup finely chopped yellow onion

2 tsp baking powder

½ tsp sea salt

2 eggs, beaten

Preheat oven to 350°F. Grease a 7 x 11-inch baking dish with cooking spray and set aside.

Place 1 cup of the corn in a large bowl and set aside. Purée remaining corn in a food processor until fairly smooth and pour into the bowl with the corn. Stir in melted Earth Balance, coconut milk, cornmeal, onion, baking powder, sea salt, and eggs and transfer to prepared dish. Bake for 50 minutes or until golden brown.

Millet Caprese Salad

Serves 4

This may not be the typical Caprese salad with sliced fresh mozzarella, but the flavors are all there. I add extra basil and some smooth cashew nut cheese when I am craving indulgence. This salad is wonderful alone or accompanied with some sliced chicken, or white beans if seeking a vegetarian option.

1 cup millet

2 ½ cups vegetable broth

1 Tbsp finely chopped fresh basil

1 tomato, diced

2 Tbsp lemon juice

1 small onion, finely chopped

¼ cup golden raisins, soaked for 10 minutes and drained

2 celery ribs, finely chopped

1 medium seedless cucumber, finely chopped

Extra virgin olive oil

In a large non-stick skillet, toast millet over high heat, shaking pan often to prevent scorching. Continue until grains begin to pop and becomes fragrant about 3 to 4 minutes, but do not burn. Transfer to a medium saucepan.

Add broth to toasted millet. Cover and bring to a boil; reduce heat to low. Cook 35 minutes. Uncover and cook 5 minutes longer. Remove millet from heat. Fluff with a fork and let cool for 10 to 15 minutes.

In a serving bowl, gently blend millet with basil, tomatoes, lemon juice, onion, golden raisins, celery and cucumber. Stir to blend. Cover and refrigerate until ready to serve. Drizzle with olive oil when ready to serve.

ENTREES

Ginger Broiled Halibut

Serves 4

Sticky, sweet and a tad spicy. Not everyone likes halibut, or fish for that matter, but I have found that even those who don't like fish truly enjoy the flavors featured in this dish. The maple syrup caramelizes the halibut rendering to a crispy crust. If you are worried about broiling, grilling or pan searing the halibut will work as well.

3 Tbsp coconut aminos
2 Tbsp maple syrup
1 Tbsp coconut oil
¼ cup filtered water
2 tsp fresh grated ginger
1 clove garlic, minced
½ tsp sea salt
4 - 4oz. wild halibut fillets
¼ cup sliced green onions

Whisk together the aminos, maple syrup, oil, water, ginger, garlic, and sea salt in a baking dish. Add the fish and marinate in sauce (skin side up) for 30 minutes. Preheat broiler to high and broil fish skin side down on the top rack of the oven for 3 to 5 minutes, depending on how you like your halibut cooked. Baste once or twice while broiling. Serve topped with green onions.

Spring Pea Ensemble

Serves 4

Peas are a wonderful source of protein. In the spring when peas are fresh and delicate, this dish is an extra special delight. It is sweet, bright and popping with flavor. I use cooked quinoa because it is a nutritional powerhouse. It offers complete protein and contains all of the essential amino acids. Quinoa helps fight fatigue, is anti-inflammatory, anti-microbial and possesses anti-cancer properties. It is a wonderful source of magnesium, lysine and quercetin.

1 Tbsp extra virgin olive oil

½ cup finely chopped red onion

1 bell pepper, diced

1 zucchini, sliced into half-moons

2 cloves garlic, finely chopped

1 tsp ground chopped dried rosemary

1 tsp dried thyme

1 tsp dried oregano

½ cup canned coconut milk

1 cup peas

1 can great northern beans, drained and rinsed

1 cup quinoa, cooked in vegetable stock

1 cup baby spinach leaves

2 Tbsp fresh basil

Zest of a lemon

Sea salt and freshly ground pepper to taste

Heat olive oil in a large skillet over medium heat. Add onion, pepper, zucchini, garlic, rosemary, thyme, and oregano. Cook about 4 minutes. Add coconut milk and peas and continue cooking for another 3 minutes. Stir in beans and cooked quinoa. Add the spinach, basil, and lemon zest and stir until wilted. Season with salt and pepper and serve immediately.

Chicken Piccata

Serves 6

I have been told that I make the best chicken piccata, even when compared to the best Italian restaurants. Although I find that hard to believe, I do admit that this dish is quite tasty and delectable. If you are seeking a vegetarian version, simply use pressed organic extra firm tofu for the chicken.

2 boneless and skinless chicken breasts, butterflied, pounded thin and sliced into cutlets

Sea salt and freshly ground black pepper

Sweet rice flour, for dredging

6 Tbsp + 2 Tbsp Earth Balance soy free spread

6 Tbsp extra virgin olive oil

½ cup fresh lemon juice

½ cup organic low sodium chicken broth (or vegetable broth if using tofu)

½ tsp sea salt

¼ tsp black pepper

1 small jar brined capers, drained

2-3 Tbsp fresh chopped parsley

1 sliced lemon

Season chicken with salt and pepper. Dredge chicken in the sweet rice flour and shake off excess flour.

In a large skillet over medium high heat, add 2 Tbsp Earth Balance and 2 Tbsp olive oil and cook until it sizzles lightly. Add 2 pieces of chicken, being careful not to overcrowd the pan, and cook for 3 minutes. When chicken is browned, flip over and cook other side for 3 minutes. Remove and transfer to plate. Repeat with remaining chicken being sure to add Earth Balance and olive oil each time prior to sautéing.

When all the chicken has been prepared, add the lemon juice and broth to the pan. Bring to a boil and whisk to scrape up the browned bits on the bottom of the plan. Add salt and pepper. Return chicken to the pan and simmer over low heat for 3 minutes. Stir in capers and simmer for 3 minutes more. Remove chicken and add 2 Tbsp Earth Balance to pan; whisking to create sauce. Strain the sauce and pour over the chicken. Garnish with parsley and lemon slices.

Salmon Loaf

Serves 4

Canned salmon is extremely affordable and even the tightest budget can work canned salmon into the weekly meal plan. Wild caught salmon poses little mercury risk, decreases inflammation, and is one of the richest sources of Omega 3 fatty acids. This recipe can also be formed into patties for the salmon burger fans out there or placed in muffin cups.

2 Tbsp extra virgin olive oil

½ cup green peppers, finely diced

½ cup onion, finely diced

2 Tbsp lemon juice

1 tsp dried dill

1 ½ cups low sodium wild caught canned salmon

1 cup steel cut oats

1 tsp sea salt

½ tsp black pepper

1 cup coconut milk

2 Tbsp chia seed combined with 6 Tbsp warm water

Fresh dill, garnish

Lemon slices, garnish

Preheat oven to 350°F.

Sauté peppers and onions in olive oil until tender. Remove from heat and stir in lemon juice and dried dill. In a large bowl, add the sautéed veggies to the remaining ingredients and mix until well combined. Pour into a greased 8" loaf pan and bake for 40 minutes until golden. Serve with fresh dill and lemons, if desired.

Sweet Apricot Turkey Meatballs

Serves 4

I feel that a sweet version of meatballs permits me to have them for breakfast, lunch or dinner. I prepare several batches of these and then freeze them so I can pull out a few at a time for a speedy snack. I generally serve the meatballs with eggs and fresh fruit or zucchini noodles and cashew cream.

2 Tbsp rice bran oil

1 apple, grated

2 Tbsp Dijon mustard

1 lb. ground turkey breast

½ cup apricot fruit spread

½ cup gluten free bread crumbs

1 Tbsp chia seed mixed with 3 Tbsp warm water

½ cup chopped spinach, defrosted and drained of all excess water

Pinch nutmeg

Sea salt & pepper to taste

Preheat oven to 400°F.

Knead all ingredients together in a large bowl. Form into balls. Heat oil over medium heat and add meatballs being careful not to overcrowd the pan. Cook, turning frequently to brown the meatballs on all sides. Place browned meatballs on a cookie sheet and bake for 15 minutes, or until cooked through.

Pumpkin Pizza

Makes 1 pizza

My clients who follow a tomato-free diet often tell me that they miss pizza the most, even more than spaghetti and meatballs. Pumpkin makes a fantastic substitute for tomato in many dishes, when paired with the right seasonings. The caramelized onions lend a bit of sweetness to the earthy sage leaves, yet there is a subtle heat from the red pepper flakes. Topped with chicken or turkey sausage, this pizza is most certain to please any pizza pie fantastic.

1 recipe for Yeasted Pizza Crust (see Extras)

¾ cup canned pumpkin

2 tsp dried sage

½ tsp pink Himalayan salt

Pinch red pepper flakes

½ tsp organic light brown sugar

½ cup vegan mozzarella style cheese

¼ cup walnut halves

¼ cup balsamic caramelized onions (recipe below)

½ cup roasted red peppers, drained and diced

1 link mild Italian chicken or turkey sausage

¼ cup fresh basil, chiffonade

6 fresh sage leaves

2 tsp balsamic glaze

Preheat oven to 450°F.

Roll out pizza crust and place on pizza pan. Bake for 5 minutes. Remove from oven and set aside.

Combine pumpkin, dried sage, salt, red pepper flakes, and brown sugar in medium bowl, stirring well. Spread onto pizza crust and sprinkle with cheese. Add the walnuts, onions, peppers, sausage, basil and sage leaves and drizzle with balsamic glaze. Bake for 15 to 20 minutes or until cheese is melted and crust is cooked through.

Caramelized Onions

1 Tbsp grapeseed oil

1 small yellow onion, halved and sliced

2 tsp balsamic vinegar

Pinch sea salt

Heat oil in a non-stick or cast iron skillet over medium low heat. When oil is hot, add the onions and a pinch of sea salt and slowly cook the onions for about 15 to 20 minutes. When the onions turn golden, add the balsamic vinegar and stir. Cook over low heat for about 5 more minutes until mixture is thick and brown. Store leftovers in a jar in the fridge for up to a week.

Bistro Chicken Salad

Serves 4

Your friends will rave over this humble chicken salad. It is as delectable as the variety you find at the specialty food shops, if not better. This salad is extremely versatile and can be adapted using any ingredients you have on hand.

2 cups cooked chicken, diced or shredded

¼ cup grated carrots

2 stalks celery, chopped

4 green onions, chopped

¼ cup grapes, sliced in half

¼ cup halved pecans

⅓ cup mayonnaise (can use light, but the fat is usually replaced with sugar)

2 Tbsp plain unsweetened coconut milk yogurt

1 tsp poppy seeds

Salt and pepper, to taste

Combine all ingredients and mix well. Season to taste.

Variations:

Curried Chicken Salad: Omit poppy seeds, grapes and pecans. Add mango chutney, diced apple, dried golden raisins or chopped apricots, green peas and season with curry powder to taste.

Oriental Chicken Salad: Omit poppy seeds, grapes and pecans. Add ½ cup each drained, chopped water chestnuts, chopped mandarin oranges, sliced almonds, ¼ tsp toasted sesame oil, ½ tsp gluten free tamari to taste.

Honey Mustard Chicken Salad: Omit poppy seeds, grapes and pecans. Blend in 2 tsp Dijon mustard and 1 Tbsp honey into mayonnaise. Add chopped cashews, diced dried apricots, dried thyme and tarragon to taste.

Cherry Rice Skillet

Serves 4

If you love cherries, you will love this dish. It has the perfect blend of sweet and savory with a nice bit of crunch from the celery. This entrée is packed with protein and is full of antioxidants and helps fight inflammation.

1 Tbsp coconut oil
½ cup onion, chopped
½ cup celery, chopped
½ cup acorn or butternut squash, small dice
1 tsp dried thyme
1 tsp dried marjoram
½ tsp ground black pepper
¼ cup chicken stock
½ cup dried tart cherries
¼ cup walnuts, chopped
2 cups cooked brown rice
2 cups cooked diced chicken
Pinch sea salt to taste

Heat coconut oil in a medium saucepan over medium high heat. Add onion, celery, squash, thyme, marjoram, and black pepper. Cook for about 10 minutes or until vegetables are softened. Add the stock, cherries, walnuts, rice and chicken, and cook until heated through and stock has evaporated. Season with sea salt to taste.

Honey Balsamic Chicken

Serves 4

We do not eat a lot of red meat in our household, so devising new chicken dishes is imperative. This dish reminds me of the sticky chicken dishes that you can find at some Asian restaurants, but with an Italian twist. It is important to be certain to use balsamic vinegar that has been aged for ten years or longer for an extra depth.

4 boneless chicken thighs

Sea salt and pepper, to taste

1 Tbsp extra virgin olive oil

½ medium onion, sliced

1 garlic clove, minced

¼ cup red wine

2 Tbsp balsamic vinegar

1 Tbsp honey

¼ cup roasted red peppers, drained and chopped

1 Tbsp dried Italian herb blend

Season chicken thighs to taste with salt and pepper. Heat oil in a skillet over medium-high heat and brown chicken thighs for 3 minutes per side. Remove chicken from pan and set aside. Add the onions and sauté until they are soft and translucent. Add the garlic and sauté for one minute, stirring to ensure the garlic doesn't burn.

Remove the pan from the heat and deglaze the pan with the red wine and scrape up any browned bits that have stuck to the bottom of the pan. Return the pan to the heat and add the balsamic vinegar, honey, roasted red peppers and Italian herbs. Simmer for 2 minutes. Return the chicken thighs to the pan and cook for an additional 5 minutes or until chicken thighs are cooked through and juices run clear.

Vegetarian Stuffed Peppers

Serves 4

My mom used to make stuffed peppers and I vividly remember eating all the filling and leaving the poor green pepper behind. I figured out years ago that I do not care for green peppers, yet I am keen on red, yellow and orange bell peppers. The stuffing can also be used in cabbage leaves or in the cavity of a seeded acorn squash. You can also make these in a Crockpot by adding a few inches of vegetable stock at the bottom with the pasta sauce before adding in the peppers. Simply cook on low for 2 to 3 hours and voila!

4 large rainbow bell peppers, cap end cut off and diced, and seeds removed

2 Tbsp extra virgin olive oil

½ cup onion, diced

½ cup celery, sliced thin

1 clove garlic, minced

2 cans lentils, drained

1 can low-sodium tomato sauce

1 cup diced tomatoes

1 Tbsp dried oregano

1 Tbsp dried basil

1 tsp ground fennel

½ tsp sea salt

¼ tsp ground black pepper

2 cups cooked quinoa or brown rice

¼ cup nutritional yeast

1 small jar favorite pasta sauce, divided

½ cup vegan shredded mozzarella cheese

Preheat oven to 350°F.

Cut tops off peppers; remove seeds and membranes. Chop edible part of tops and set aside. Place the peppers in a large pot and cover with salted water. Bring to a boil. Reduce heat to a simmer and cook for 5 to 7 minutes. Drain peppers and set aside.

Meanwhile, heat olive oil and in a large skillet over medium heat until hot. Sauté reserved chopped bell pepper tops, onion, celery and garlic for about 5 minutes, or until vegetables are tender. Stir in lentils, tomato sauce, diced tomatoes, oregano, basil, fennel, salt and pepper. Simmer for about 10 minutes.

Gently fold in cooked quinoa and nutritional yeast. Pour half of the pasta sauce into bottom of baking dish. Stuff peppers with lentil mixture and place in the baking dish on top of the pasta sauce. Pour remaining tomato mixture over the stuffed peppers and top with cheese. Cover and bake for 1 hour. Remove cover and bake another 10 to 15 minutes.

English Pot Roast

Serves 8

My husband loves pot roast, especially my recipe. Not only does it make him happy, it is very easy to make, thanks to the trusty slow cooker. Typically, fatty cuts of meat produce more flavor, however, since the round roast is cooked in the slow cooker, the beef remains juicy, rich and hearty.

2 Tbsp organic cornstarch

2 Tbsp avocado oil

3 to 4 lbs. grass fed beef or bison round roast

6 large stalks celery, chopped

3 cups baby carrots

1 large onion, cubed

1 lb. red potatoes, quartered

1 large turnip, cubed

1 bay leaf

2 cups beef stock

1 Tbsp minced garlic

1 tsp pink Himalayan salt

1 tsp pepper

Place cornstarch in large zip lock bag and add roast, shaking to coat. Remove roast from bag and sear on all sides in avocado oil in large pot. Remove and set aside.

Place the celery, carrots, onion, potatoes, turnip, and bay leaf, at the bottom of a slow cooker. Pour in beef stock. Add the roast to the crockpot, placing on top of veggies. Rub minced garlic onto top of roast, and sprinkle with salt and pepper.

Cook on low for 6 to 8 hours or until meat easily flakes. Remove bay leaf before serving.

Better Bean Loaf

Serves 3

This loaf recipe is a spin on meatloaf for your vegetarian friends, or for when you are trying to cut back on meat. The combination of spices, beans, and potato make for a very happy palate. Sweet potatoes are full of beta carotene, potassium, vitamin B6 and vitamin C. In addition, they are a fantastic choice for balancing the endocrine system, and aiding those with night blindness and/or cataracts.

1 ½ cup canned chickpeas, drained and rinsed

½ cup cooked peas

½ cup onions, chopped

1 Tbsp tomato paste (optional)

1 tsp cumin

1 tsp dried oregano

1 tsp dried thyme

½ tsp sea salt

¼ cup extra virgin olive oil

2 cups boiled sweet potato, mashed

½ cup cashews, chopped

Coconut oil, to grease pan

Preheat oven to 350°F.

Sauté the chickpeas, peas, onions, tomato paste, cumin, oregano, thyme, and sea salt in the oil in a large saucepan over medium heat until softened. Scoop the chickpea mixture into a food processor and run until paste forms. Add in mashed sweet potatoes and cashews and pulse 2 or 3 times. Spread the bean mixture into a greased loaf pan and bake for 45 minutes. Let cool slightly before serving.

Simple Fish Tacos with Mango & Blueberry Salsa

Serves 4

Fish Tacos are a wonderful way to create a protein-rich meal that does not weigh you down. This dish is perfect for a hot summer night when you can count on the colorful and vibrant salsa to cool you down.

Salsa:

½ cup blueberries

½ cup mango, small dice

2 Tbsp red onion, finely chopped

2 Tbsp red bell pepper, finely chopped

1 Tbsp fresh cilantro

1 Tbsp fresh lime juice

½ tsp jalapeño, seeded and finely chopped

1-2 tsp raw honey

Sea salt to taste

Fish:

1 ½ lbs. fresh white fish filets (cod, halibut, flounder, grouper, haddock, etc.)

2 Tbsp extra virgin olive oil

½ tsp sea salt or favorite seafood seasoning

¼ tsp lemon pepper

Gluten free tortillas (corn, rice, etc.)

Cashew cream, for garnish (see Extras)

Combine all salsa ingredients in bowl, crush fruit slightly and stir. Set aside to steep.

Rub fish lightly with olive oil and sprinkle with sea salt and pepper. Heat a non-stick skillet over medium high heat. Add fish and cook for 3 to 4 minutes, and then turn over, cooking for 2 to 3 minutes longer. Remove from heat.

Compile tacos by placing the fish in a soft corn or gluten free tortilla, top with salsa and drizzle with cashew cream.

Chicken Pot Pie

Serves 6

What is it about Chicken Pot Pie that makes everyone so happy? It is perhaps the most comforting dish in my opinion. Although I grew up on the frozen varieties, I find making homemade pot pie represents love in a pie dish. There is something about cooking it from scratch that makes it extra special on any cool night.

5 Tbsp extra virgin olive oil

2 medium shallots, diced

3 medium celery stalks, cut on the diagonal into ¼" thick slices

4 medium carrots, diced into ½" cubes

1 garlic clove, minced

½ tsp coarse sea salt

¼ tsp freshly ground pepper

2 cups chicken stock, divided

2 Tbsp arrowroot

2 cups diced cooked chicken

1 cup slightly thawed frozen peas

¼ cup coarsely chopped fresh flat-leaf parsley, plus more for garnish

1 tsp finely chopped fresh tarragon

Prepared pie crust (see Extras)

Earth Balance soy free spread, melted (for brushing)

Preheat oven to 400°F.

Heat olive oil in a medium saucepan over medium heat. Add shallots, celery, carrots, garlic, salt and pepper and sauté 3 minutes. Add 1 ½ cups stock. Whisk remaining ½ cup stock into the arrowroot in a small bowl. Whisk this into shallot mixture and bring to a gentle boil, whisking constantly until mixture begins to thicken. Reduce heat to a simmer and cook for 5 minutes, whisking occasionally.

Add in chicken and cook until heated through. Remove from heat and stir in peas, chopped parsley and tarragon. Pour mixture into prepared piecrust. Top with remaining scattered pieces of crust. Brush with melted Earth Balance and bake for 30 minutes or until bubbly and golden brown.

Simple Veggie Burgers

Makes 12 – 3" burgers

The crunch of this burger makes it a real treat and reminds me of the chicken patties I used to consume when money was tight. The thought makes me shudder! These veggie burgers are meatless, do not contain GMOs and are full of fiber and protein to fuel your day.

½ cup raw kale

¼ cup shredded zucchini

¼ cup raw walnuts

¼ cup gluten free quick oats

1 shallot, minced

2 Tbsp nutritional yeast flakes

1 Tbsp Dijon mustard

1 Tbsp garlic paste

2 tsp dried thyme

1 tsp Greek seasoning

1 tsp sea salt

¼ tsp black pepper

1 can cannellini beans, drained and rinsed

1 cup cooked brown rice

Preheat oven to 350°F.

Add the kale, zucchini, walnuts, oats, and shallot to a food processor and pulse to combine. Add in nutritional yeast, mustard, garlic paste, thyme, Greek seasoning, salt and pepper and pulse a few times. Add beans and pulse until mixture starts to pull together. Add rice and pulse two to three times, making sure to keep some rice whole.

Remove mixture from food processor and form into patties. Place on a greased cookie sheet and bake for 20 minutes. Flip the burgers and bake for 15 more minutes or until golden brown and crispy on the edges.

Homemade Sweet Potato Gnocchi

Makes 4 servings

Just about the time I tried gnocchi and fell in love with it, I found out I had a gluten intolerance. Although there are a few gluten free gnocchi products in the natural food stores today, they are extremely pricey considering the amount you receive in the package. I made it a mission to create my own recipe and found that I am extremely fond of this sweet potato version.

2 cups sweet potatoes, boiled and mashed
1 ¼ cup superfine brown rice flour plus more for dusting
½ tsp sea salt

Boil potatoes in large pot. Drain and allow to cool.

Next, process the potatoes, flour and see salt in the bowl of a food processor and pulse until crumbly. Dust a clean surface with flour. Pour the sweet potato mixture on to the surface. Divide the dough in half and roll each piece into a thin rope. You may add more flour if it is too sticky. Cut into 1" pieces and gently apply the tines of a fork, pressing gently and rolling each gnocchi to make tine marks. Drop gnocchi in boiling water and cook until they float, about 4 or 5 minutes. Drain and serve warm with sage sauce.

Sauce:
2 Tbsp Earth Balance soy free spread
8 fresh sage leaves
1 Tbsp tapioca starch whisked into ¼ cup plain coconut creamer
½ tsp sea salt
¼ tsp black pepper
Dash nutmeg

Melt the Earth Balance in a skillet over medium-high heat. Add the sage and cook until crispy. Add in creamer mixture, sea salt, pepper, and nutmeg. Continue to cook, whisking constantly, until thickened. Toss with cooked gnocchi.

Penne Pasta with Clever Creamy Corn Sauce

Serves 6-8

Velvety rich, with a sunny yellow hue that reminds me of the Sun. It is unapologetically indulgent and decadent.

4 cups frozen organic corn, thawed (or fresh is best), divided

1 ½ cups organic chicken stock

1 Tbsp extra virgin olive oil

5 slices turkey bacon, chopped

½ tsp sea salt

¼ tsp ground black pepper

3 leeks, washed and thinly sliced (use only the whites)

4 cloves garlic, minced

1 Tbsp fresh thyme

⅓ cup fresh basil, chiffonade

1 lb. gluten free penne pasta, cooked 2 minutes less than package instructions

2 Tbsp Earth Balance spread

Vegan parmesan, if desired

Chopped fresh parsley, for garnish

Puree 2 cups of corn with chicken stock in blender. Set aside.

In a sauté pan, add olive oil and bacon and cook to crisp. Add the remaining 2 cups of corn kernels, sea salt and pepper and cook, stirring occasionally, for 2 to 4 minutes. Stir in leeks, garlic, thyme, and basil and cook 2 minutes longer. Stir in corn puree and heat through over low heat. Toss together with Earth Balance, pasta and vegan parmesan until well coated. Sprinkle with parsley and serve.

Stuffed Turkey

Serves 2-3

Stuffed turkey breast can be sophisticated when the right ingredients are used. My Stuffed Turkey pairs tart dried cranberries, nutty winter squash and earthy quinoa. It is low in calories, rich in protein and highly nutritive. This makes a distinctive entrée perfect for any special occasion.

4 Tbsp extra virgin olive oil, divided

1 small onion, diced

1 clove garlic

1 Tbsp dried rosemary

2 Tbsp plus ¼ cup turkey stock

4 cups raw spinach

1 cup cooked quinoa

1 cup cooked butternut squash, finely diced

⅓ cup fruit juice sweetened dried cranberries

2 boneless, skinless turkey breasts

Salt and pepper to taste

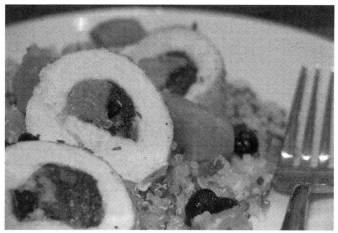

Preheat oven to 350°F.

In a large skillet, sauté the onions, garlic and rosemary in 2 tablespoons olive oil until the onions are translucent. Deglaze the pan with stock, scraping up any bits on the bottom of the pan. Pour into a bowl and stir in spinach, quinoa, butternut squash and cranberries.

Butterfly the turkey breast horizontally and pound between parchment paper or plastic wrap. Season the turkey breast with salt and pepper and spoon the quinoa mixture into each breast. Roll to seal and fasten with toothpicks. Place the rolled turkey breasts in a baking dish and drizzle with the remaining olive oil. Cover and bake for 25 minutes or until turkey is cooked through.

Vegetable Empanadas

Makes 4 empanadas

Portable hand pies that are stuffed with beans and veggies are genius. Sometimes I use white beans, sundried tomatoes and roasted red peppers for an Italian spin, with a side of marinara for dipping. Whatever style you choose, your family will love what you have to offer.

1 cup refried beans

1 Tbsp diced chilies

1 tsp cumin

1 cup vegan shredded cheddar or pepper jack cheese, divided

½ cup onion, diced

½ cup pepper, diced

2 Tbsp Earth Balance soy free spread

2 Tbsp non-dairy milk

1 Tbsp flaxseed mixed with 3 Tbsp warm water

1 tsp baking soda

1 tsp lemon juice

1 cup organic masa harina (corn flour)

½ tsp xanthan gum

½ tsp sea salt

1 Tbsp melted Earth Balance soy free spread

Salsa, Cashew Cream, fresh cilantro, and Guacamole for garnish (see Extras)

Preheat oven to 400°F.

In a small bowl, mix beans together with chilies and cumin. Set aside.

With a hand mixer, cream together ½ the cheese, onion, pepper, Earth Balance, milk and flaxseed mixture until well combined. Next, beat in the baking soda and lemon juice. Finally, on low speed, add in the corn flour, xanthan gum, and sea salt, mixing until a loose ball forms.

Remove the dough and place onto a surface sprinkled with masa. Divide the dough into four pieces and roll each piece into a ball. Using a rolling pin, roll each ball to ¼" thickness. Place each circle onto a parchment lined baking sheet. Spoon ¼ cup of the bean mixture into the bottom half of the center of dough and top with cheese. Fold in half and press together to form pocket. Seal the edges using the tines of a fork and slit each pocket with a knife. Brush the pockets with Earth Balance and bake 15 to 18 minutes or until golden. Serve with salsa, cashew cream, fresh cilantro and guacamole.

Ratatouille

Serves 4

Ratatouille makes an elegant yet simple supper that is delicious when served over grilled polenta and drizzled with cashew cream. It is an excellent use of summer vegetables and fills the air with a deep and rich aroma.   Leftovers are as delicious and are fantastic for breakfast with a poached egg on top.

¼ cup extra virgin olive oil

2 ½ cups eggplant, chopped

1 cup sliced onion

2 cups sliced red peppers

2 cups zucchini, chopped

2 cloves crushed garlic

2 cups diced tomatoes

2 Tbsp chopped Kalamata olives

1 Tbsp Italian seasoning

2 cups pasta sauce

Heat a large skillet over medium high heat. Add olive oil and add the eggplant, onions, peppers, zucchini, garlic, and tomatoes. Cook for 6 minutes, stirring occasionally. Add the olives, Italian seasoning and pasta sauce and simmer until vegetables are tender. Serve warm.

Seductive Pasta

Serves 6

This recipe is economical and a cinch to make. The sauce is divine with its rich and velvety consistency and has a slight, yet impeccable acidity from the artichokes. The wine adds perkiness and the raisins add a sweet note. I recommend adding sliced sundried tomato chicken sausage for extra verve.

4 Tbsp extra virgin olive oil

4 cloves fresh garlic, minced

1 – 10oz. package frozen artichoke hearts, thawed and chopped

½ cup golden raisins

2 cups baby spinach

Pinch red pepper flakes

2 Tbsp dry white wine

1 lb. brown rice penne pasta, cooked 1 to 2 minutes less than package instructions

½ cup pecan pieces

½ cup vegan mozzarella cheese

¼ cup fresh basil chiffonade

Sea salt & freshly ground pepper, to taste

Heat the olive oil over medium heat in a large skillet, and add the garlic; stir just until the garlic begins to soften and turn golden. Add the chopped artichokes and stir. When the artichokes soften, add the raisins, spinach, red pepper flakes and the wine.

Toss the cooked pasta into the artichoke mixture. Stir in the pecans, cheese, and basil. Season with sea salt and freshly ground pepper, to taste. Serve immediately.

Vegan Spinach Enchiladas

Serves 3

Mexican cuisine is very popular and enjoyed by many. Even before avoiding dairy, I always found the fatty sauces and gobs of cheese overpowering. Spinach enchiladas are light in calories and exceptional in taste. This dish never gets old in our family.

1 Tbsp extra virgin olive oil

1 small red onion, chopped

1 red bell pepper, diced

2 cloves garlic, minced

1 - 10 oz. package frozen organic spinach

½ cup shredded zucchini

1 cup cooked quinoa

1 can no salt added black beans, drained and rinsed

2 tomatoes, chopped

1 can green chilies, drained

½ tsp chili powder

½ tsp ground cumin

1 tsp dried Mexican oregano

1 cup salsa

6 soft corn tortillas

1 jar enchilada sauce

¾ cup vegan shredded mozzarella cheese

Preheat oven to 350°F.

Heat oil in a large skillet over medium heat. Sauté the onion, red pepper and garlic, stirring often. Add spinach, zucchini, quinoa, beans, tomatoes, chilies, chili powder, cumin, oregano, and salsa and cook until heated through. Pour one third of the sauce in bottom of baking dish. Divide filling among tortillas, roll and place in baking dish with seam side down. Top with remaining salsa and sprinkle with cheese. Bake for about 25 minutes until bubbly.

Sarah's Lasagna

Makes 6 -8 servings

This recipe took years to develop and although I try to keep my recipes soy free, I have found that using a nut-based ricotta alternative makes the dish too heavy. Small amounts of organic, sprouted tofu are not harmful if used sparingly, and I believe this dish makes the best use of the tofu. Lasagna is a several step process and this recipe is no different. This dish is to die for!

2 Tbsp extra virgin olive oil

1 lb. chicken Italian sausage (optional)

White Sauce (Béchamel):

2 Tbsp sweet rice flour

2 Tbsp extra virgin olive oil

2 cups coconut milk, or other non-dairy milk

1 tsp garlic powder

1 tsp sea salt

½ tsp ground white pepper

½ tsp red pepper flakes (optional)

2 cups frozen shredded spinach or kale, defrosted and squeezed dry

Tofu Ricotta Mixture:

1 container extra firm organic tofu (not aseptic container, preferably sprouted)

3 garlic cloves, minced

1 package vegan mozzarella shredded cheese

1 ½ Tbsp Italian herb blend

½ tsp sea salt

1 jar pasta sauce

½ package boxed brown rice lasagna noodles, cooked according to package instructions

Preheat oven to 375°F.

Brown sausage in 2 Tbsp olive oil. Set aside when cooked through.

In another pan, prepare the white sauce by combining flour and olive oil in large pan over medium high heat. Cook for 1 minute, and whisk in coconut milk. Once thickened, stir in garlic powder, sea salt, white pepper, and red pepper flakes. Stir in spinach or kale. Set aside.

In medium bowl, combine tofu, garlic and salt and break apart using a fork until a ricotta cheese texture is reached. Stir in about 1 cup of the mozzarella cheese, Italian herb blend, and sea salt.

In baking dish, or bread loaf pan, pour ¼ cup of pasta sauce on bottom. Lay a single layer of lasagna noodles over the pasta sauce. Next, spread ¼ cup of the tofu mixture and then spread ¼ cup of the béchamel over the tofu mixture. Next, lay a single layer of lasagna noodles, then spread ¼ cup pasta sauce over the noodles and sprinkle ½ of the sausage on top. Repeat layers. Finally, top with one more layer of noodles, the remaining pasta sauce and then the remaining cheese. Sprinkle the top with dried basil and oregano. Bake for about 30 minutes, or until bubbly and golden brown on top. Remove from oven and allow to sit for 15 minutes before serving.

EXTRAS

Coconut Bacon

Serves 15

This recipe sounds outlandish, but coconut bacon has the same smoky taste found in the animal protein versions. I sprinkle Coconut Bacon over salads or over pasta dishes (think pasta carbonara). It is zany and so yummy.

3 ½ cups large flaked unsweetened coconut

2 Tbsp gluten free liquid smoke

1 Tbsp coconut aminos

1 Tbsp maple syrup

1 Tbsp water

1 tsp apple cider vinegar

1 tsp coconut oil, liquid

½ tsp ground pepper

Pinch sea salt

Preheat oven to 325°F.

Combine all ingredients in a medium bowl and stir to coat. Allow to sit 5 minutes, and stir again. Wait 5 more minutes, then strain and pour onto a non-stick baking sheet. Bake for 20 minutes, flipping regularly until crispy and golden.

Flour Blends

Below you will find recipes for a variety of flour blends that you can mix in advance and store in glass jars in the pantry for convenience.

<u>All Purpose Blend</u>
1 cup superfine brown rice flour
1 cup white rice flour
½ cup sorghum or millet flour
½ cup tapioca flour
½ cup potato starch

For breads, muffins, and soft cookies, add 1 tsp xanthan, guar gum, or unflavored gelatin, if desired, per 2 cups of All Purpose Blend.

For a self-rising flour blend, add 1 ½ tsp of baking powder and ¼ tsp sea salt per 1 cup of All Purpose Blend.

<u>Cake Flour Blend</u>
1 ½ cups superfine white rice flour
½ cup potato starch
½ cup tapioca starch
½ cup millet flour
1 tsp baking powder
1 tsp baking soda
1 tsp xanthan gum

Whole Grain Blend

1 cup superfine brown rice flour

1 cup sorghum or millet flour

½ cup millet flour

½ cup gluten free oat flour

½ cup teff flour

½ cup buckwheat flour

Grain Free Blend

2 cups almond flour

1 cup coconut flour

½ cup ground flaxseed or ground chia seed

½ cup psyllium powder

High Fiber Blend

1 ½ cup almond flour

1 cup sweet potato flour

½ cup coconut flour

½ cup ground flaxseed

½ cup psyllium powder

Dressings

Salad dressings are extremely easy to make, are inexpensive and taste so much better than the store bought brands. I like to experiment with flavors by using flavored vinegars, sea salts or oils, fresh herbs and fruits of the season. I am certain these recipes will have you making your own dressings in no time!

Balsamic Vinaigrette

½ cup balsamic vinegar

1 Tbsp Dijon mustard

2 cloves garlic

1 tsp sea salt

½ tsp black pepper

¼ cup extra virgin olive oil

¼ cup grape seed oil

¼ cup almond oil

Place all ingredients except the oils into a blender and process until smooth. With the blender running, slowly pour in the oils. Store dressing in the fridge for up to 5 days.

Pumpkin Maple Salad Dressing

½ cup pumpkin puree

6 Tbsp apple cider

¼ cup raw apple cider vinegar

¼ cup plain coconut milk yogurt

¼ cup avocado oil

2 Tbsp maple syrup

1 Tbsp almond butter

1 Tbsp Dijon mustard

1 ½ tsp dried sage

1 tsp dried thyme

¾ tsp garlic powder

¾ tsp onion powder

¾ tsp sea salt

¼ tsp black pepper

Put all ingredients in a blender and run until thick and creamy. Keep refrigerated until ready to use.

Vegan Caesar Dressing

¼ cup raw cashews, soaked for 1 hour

2 Tbsp raw pine nuts, macadamia nuts or sunflower seeds, soaked for 1 hour

3 Tbsp apple cider vinegar

1 Tbsp extra virgin olive oil

2 small cloves garlic

1 tsp brown rice miso paste

1 tsp dulse flakes

½ tsp sea salt

1 packet stevia

¼ cup water (more as needed)

½ tsp black pepper

Add all the ingredients and purée until very smooth. Add the reserved water a little bit at a time until the desired consistency is reached. Store dressing in the fridge for up to 5 days.

Tahini Dressing

½ cup tahini

½ cup water

¼ cup lemon juice

1 Tbsp raw honey

2 cloves garlic

2 tsp dried thyme

2 tsp dried tarragon

¾ tsp sea salt

Blend ingredients together until smooth. Add additional water, 1 Tbsp at a time, for a thinner dressing. Store dressing in the fridge for up to 5 days. Stir or shake if dressing separates.

Italian Dressing

¼ cup grape seed oil

¼ cup red wine vinegar

¼ cup apple cider vinegar

2 Tbsp water

1 very small garlic clove, minced

½ small shallot, minced

1 tsp dried thyme

1 tsp dried parsley

1 tsp dried basil

1 packet stevia

Celery seed, sea salt and pepper to taste

In a small bowl, whisk together all ingredients. Store dressing in the fridge for up to 5 days.

Dairy free Ranch Dressing

¼ cup vegan mayonnaise

1 tablespoon lemon juice, fresh squeezed

1 clove garlic, minced

½ tsp dried parsley

¼ tsp dried thyme

⅛ tsp minced scallions

Sea salt and pepper to taste

Combine all ingredients in a small bowl. Whisk well. Store dressing in the fridge for up to 5 days.

Apple Cider Vinaigrette

½ cup apple cider vinegar

¼ cup apple cider

2 Tbsp maple syrup

2 tsp sea salt

1 tsp cracked black pepper

½ tsp cayenne pepper

1 tsp ground cinnamon

2 cups avocado oil

Combine all ingredients except oil in blender. Once mixture has combined, stream in the oil with blender running until thick and smooth. Store dressing in the fridge for up to 5 days.

Orange Cardamom Vinaigrette

4 small shallot, minced

2 pitted medjool dates

½ cup citrus flavored vinegar

¼ cup raw honey

¼ cup orange juice

3 Tbsp Dijon mustard

1 tsp sea salt, more to taste

½ tsp orange essential oil

½ tsp ground cardamom

¼ tsp ground white pepper

½ cup grape seed oil

Combine the shallot, pitted dates and vinegar in high speed blender. Blend on high until smooth and dates have broken down. Add in all remaining ingredients except oil in blender. Once mixture has combined, stream in the oil with blender running until thick and smooth. Store dressing in the fridge for up to 5 days.

Strawberry Basil Vinaigrette

½ cup fresh or frozen raspberries

¼ cup water

¼ cup apple cider vinegar

1 tsp sea salt

2 Tbsp honey

5 basil leaves

¾ cup extra virgin olive oil

Combine all ingredients except oil in blender. Once mixture has combined, stream in the oil with blender running until thick and smooth. Store dressing in the fridge for up to 5 days.

Date Paste

Makes approximately 1 pint

Using date paste instead of other liquid sweeteners is a fantastic way to increase your fiber intake with a healthy punch of zinc and iron. I love to use a teaspoon or two stirred into my gluten free steel cut oats for a deep and dark flavor.

1 ½ cup water

1 cup soft medjool dates, pitted, soaked for 1 hour and drained

¼ tsp sea salt

1 tsp lemon juice

Blend all ingredients in high speed blender until completely smooth.

Egg Free Mayonnaise Recipes

People either love or hate mayonnaise. I created these recipes for a few friends who truly dislike the texture of mayonnaise. These recipes are a wonderful alternative for those who are vegan or have allergies to eggs. They are light in flavor and texture and are high in magnesium, a nutrient in which many people are deficient.

Avocado Mayonnaise

1 avocado

1 Tbsp lemon juice

1 tsp apple cider vinegar

1 tsp Dijon mustard

¼ tsp sea salt

⅛ tsp onion powder

2 Tbsp extra virgin olive oil

Combine all ingredients, except olive oil, in a food processor and run until chunks disappear. With the motor running, drizzle in the olive oil until mayonnaise is creamy, light in color and texture. Store in fridge for up to a week.

Tarragon Cashew Mayonnaise

1 cup raw cashews, soaked 1 hour and drained

1 small shallot

2 Tbsp fresh tarragon

1 ½ Tbsp fresh lemon juice

2 tsp apple cider vinegar

1 tsp organic sugar

1 tsp Dijon mustard

1 tsp sea salt

¼ cup extra virgin olive oil

Blend all ingredients in high speed blender, except olive oil, until smooth. With blender running, stream in the olive oil. Store in fridge for up to 8 days.

Sugar Free BBQ Sauce

When following a yeast free diet, most condiments are off-limit. Homemade BBQ sauce is naturally delicious and has unique charm that is addictive.

1 - 6 oz. can tomato paste

⅔ cup water

2 Tbsp coconut aminos

1 ½ tsp chili powder

1 tsp dry mustard

1 tsp sea salt

2 tsp lemon juice

2 Tbsp raw apple cider vinegar

1 tsp crushed garlic

2 Tbsp minced onion

4 Tbsp yacon syrup

⅛ tsp gluten free liquid smoke

1 packet stevia

Combine all ingredients in food processor or blender and blend until desired consistency.

Almond Feta Cheese

Serves 10

Vegan cheeses are astonishingly delicious and this version is no different. I use this recipe to crumble atop salads or use to stuff gluten free pasta shells. It fulfills any craving for a creamy, salty and scrumptious accent to any dish.

1 cup whole blanched almonds (see note below)

¼ cup lemon juice

3 Tbsp extra virgin olive oil

1 garlic clove

1 tsp sea salt

1 probiotic capsule

½ cup water

Place almonds in medium bowl and cover with 3 inches of water. Let soak 24 hours. Drain and peel off almond skins, if using regular almonds. Rinse.

Puree almonds, lemon juice, olive oil, garlic, salt and ½ cup water in blender or food processor for 6 minutes or until really creamy. Add in probiotic and pulse 3 to 4 times.

Place a triple layer of cheesecloth in a mesh strainer and spoon almond mixture into cheesecloth Twist the top of the cheesecloth to make an orange-sized ball and secure with a twist tie. Return the ball to the strainer and place over a bowl. Chill for 12 hours.

Line baking sheet with parchment and transfer almond ball from cheesecloth. Shape into a ball and bake in oven at 325°F for 60 minutes or until top is slightly firm. Cool and chill for 2 hours. Slice into ½" chunks and bake at 350°F for 20 minutes. Cool and store in fridge for up to 1 week.

Whole Grain Dinner Rolls

Makes 8 - 3 ½" rolls

At every dinner event, there is a basket of dinner rolls. When I went gluten free, I passed the basket to my neighbor only after closing my eyes and inhaling the yeasty aroma wafting from the soft roll. Now I am free to partake in the crusty roll. They are so exquisite and mouthwatering, it is hard to tell that they are gluten free.

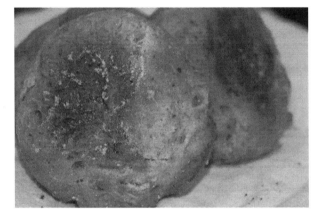

½ cup superfine brown rice flour

½ cup sorghum flour

½ cup potato starch

¼ cup tapioca starch

¼ cup millet flour

1 tsp sea salt

1 ½ tsp baking soda

1 Tbsp baking powder

¼ cup ground chia seed mixed with ¾ cup warm water

½ cup warm non-dairy milk

1 tsp apple cider vinegar

4 Tbsp avocado oil

1 Tbsp raw honey

Preheat oven to 425°F. Spray English muffin rings with coconut oil and set aside.

In a large mixing bowl, whisk together brown rice flour, sorghum flour, potato starch, tapioca starch, millet flour, sea salt, baking soda, and baking powder. Set aside.

In separate bowl, mix the chia seed mixture, milk, vinegar, oil, and honey with a hand mixer. Blend wet mixture into dry ingredients and combine until smooth. Scoop dough into prepared muffin rings. Bake in preheated oven for 20 to 25 minutes or until golden brown.

Note: If you do not have English muffin rings, you can bake inside biscuit cutters or greased muffins tins.

Sandwich Rounds

Makes 12 rounds

As a gluten free gal, I was jealous when the lower calorie thin rolls came out a few years ago. I never liked huge chunks of bread to surround my sandwich fillings, but there were no flat sandwich rolls for me to try that were safe. It motivated me to get in the kitchen and find a way to bake a gluten free sandwich round with plenty of flavor that even those who prefer white bread would love.

2 ½ cups warm water

1 package active dry yeast

1 cup superfine brown rice flour

1 cup millet flour

½ cup potato starch

½ cup tapioca starch

½ cup sorghum flour

1 tsp sea salt

½ tsp xanthan gum

2 tablespoons cornmeal (optional)

Preheat oven to 450° F.

Line a cookie sheet with parchment paper and sprinkle with the cornmeal. Set aside.

In the bowl of a stand mixer fitted with the paddle attachment, mix the water and the yeast with a fork. Allow to sit for five minutes to soften the yeast. Add the flours, salt and xanthan gum and turn the mixer on low speed until flour is all wet. Beat on high for 5 minutes.

Scoop the dough into 12 rounds on the parchment lined cookie sheet sprinkled with cornmeal. Allow to rise for about 45 minutes. Bake for 8 minutes and then add 6 to 8 cubes of ice to bottom of oven to produce steam. Bake for 12 more minutes until brown. Cool on wire rack.

HONESTLY GLUTEN FREE & DAIRY FREE

Perfect Pizza Crust

Makes 2 – 8-10" pizza crusts

Almost all pizza crusts contain yeast, yet so many people are sensitive to yeast. Although yeasted doughs produce a bubbly crust, taste is most important and this crust is delicious. The best part about making yeast free dough is that it can be prepared quickly since there is no rising time. This crust has a crispy, yet soft, texture that is the perfect foundation for homemade sauce and fresh vegetables.

½ cup millet flour

½ cup brown rice flour

½ cup potato starch

½ cup white rice flour

½ cup tapioca flour

2 Tbsp psyllium husk

½ tsp sea salt

1 ½ tsp baking powder

¾ tsp baking soda

½ tsp xanthan gum

1 cup seltzer water

¼ cup unsweetened plain coconut yogurt

2 Tbsp extra virgin olive oil

1 Tbsp apple cider vinegar

1 tsp organic sugar (optional)

Preheat oven to 375° F. In the bowl of a stand mixer, combine all dry ingredients and turn on low speed to stir flours. Add the remaining ingredients and blend on medium speed until incorporated and dough ball forms.

Scoop out onto an oiled pizza pan and using a spatula, form the dough into a thin sheet covering the pan. Bake the crust for about 15 minutes until desired crispiness.

Increase oven temp to 475°F. Top the baked crust with pizza sauce and your favorite toppings. Return pizza to oven until desired doneness, about 10 to 18 minutes.

Yeasted Pizza Dough

Makes 1 – 12" pizza crust

This is a fantastic, crispy pizza crust loaded with flavor. It is a traditional style crust that holds up well to sauces without getting soggy.

½ cup millet flour

½ cup brown rice flour

½ cup tapioca flour

2 Tbsp potato starch

1 cup seltzer water, warmed

1 ½ tsp baking powder

1 tsp yeast

1 tsp xanthan gum

1 tsp sea salt

Cornmeal

Combine all ingredients, except cornmeal in the bowl of a mixer. Run on high speed until dough is well combined. Remove and add dough to a greased bowl and let rise in a warm place for 1 hour.

Preheat oven to 475°F.

Pour dough onto floured surface and knead 2-3 times. Roll out to ½" thickness and the desired shape. Sprinkle cornmeal on parchment lined pizza pan or cookie sheet and place dough on top. Bake for 5 minutes and remove. Add sauce and toppings of choice and bake for an additional 10 to 15 minutes.

Pasta Sauce

Makes 1 ½ pints

Pasta sauce is seldom in my grocery cart because I find that even the $12 jars do not taste as good or fresh as my homemade sauce. By slowly simmering the tomatoes and seasonings together, the result is a lusciously smooth and scintillating sauce. During the tomato harvest at the end of summer, we prepare this sauce by the gallon so we have a supply to last until the next season; but we always seem to run out well beforehand.

3 Tbsp extra virgin olive oil
½ small onion, grated
2 garlic cloves, minced
3 ½ cups crushed tomatoes
2 Tbsp fresh basil
1 Tbsp fresh thyme
1 Tbsp fresh oregano
½ tsp sea salt
½ cup organic red wine (optional)

In a large saucepan, heat oil over medium high heat. Add onions and sauté until soft. Stir in minced garlic and cook for 2 minutes, careful not to burn. Stir in tomatoes and simmer for 20 minutes, or until sauce is reduces to about 2 ½ cups. Season sauce with herbs and wine and cool to room temperature. (Sauce keeps, covered and chilled, 5 days).

Pesto Recipes

Green Pesto Spread

Makes approximately 1 ½ cups

I am not a huge fan of pesto sauce on pasta, but I find it irresistible when spread on a wrap, as a garnish in hot soup or spread atop a gluten free cracker with Almond Feta Cheese. I concocted this spread to be creamy and thick yet verdant and robust in flavor.

1 bunch basil leaves

¼ cup pine nuts or raw walnuts

2 ripe avocados, pitted and peeled

2 Tbsp fresh lemon juice

3 cloves garlic

¼ cup extra virgin olive oil

Salt to taste

Freshly ground black pepper to taste

In a food processor, blend basil, pine nuts, avocados, lemon juice, and garlic. Once combined, with food processor running, drizzle in olive oil. Season with salt and pepper to taste.

Leafy Green Pesto Sauce

Makes approximately 1 cup

This version is akin to traditional pesto sauce. I incorporate a hefty dose of healthy, leafy greens and use slightly less basil so it is less bitter.

1 cup kale

1 cup spinach

¼ cup fresh basil

1 garlic clove

¼ cup pine nuts

¼ cup nutritional yeast

2 Tbsp lemon juice

¼ extra virgin olive oil

Sea salt and pepper

In a food processor, pulse kale, spinach, and basil 4 or 5 times. Add in garlic, pine nuts, nutritional yeast, and lemon juice, and run until all ingredients are combined. With motor running, drizzle in olive oil. Season with salt and pepper to taste.

Cranberry Apple Compote

Makes 4 servings

Fruit toppings can be a healthy accent to sweet or savory dishes. My cranberry apple compote takes the freshest fruits of autumn and transforms it into a thick, naturally sweet blend ideal for French toast, yogurt, ice cream or anything else you desire.

1 cup organic apple cider

4 Tbsp maple syrup

2 Tbsp organic dark brown sugar

2 Tbsp Earth Balance soy free spread, divided

2 organic apples, peeled (if desired), cored, cut into ½" pieces

2 cups fresh or thawed cranberries

Zest of an orange

Pinch sea salt

Whisk apple cider, maple syrup, and brown sugar in heavy large saucepan. Boil over high heat until reduced to 1 cup, about 15 minutes. Add 1 tablespoon Earth Balance; whisk until melted. Remove from heat.

Melt remaining Earth Balance in heavy large skillet over medium heat. Add apples; sauté 2 minutes. Add cranberries and cook until cranberries begin to pop, about 2 minutes. Stir in reduced cider mixture. Boil until reduced to syrup consistency, about 6 minutes. Add orange zest. Serve warm over ice cream, oatmeal or warm French toast.

Sarah's Raw Chocolate Fudge Sauce

Makes 12 servings

People have offered me money to obtain this recipe prior to the cookbooks release, and I have resisted the temptation knowing that the best things in life are worth the wait. This is a straightforward recipe that takes just seconds to prepare.

½ cup coconut oil

½ cup cacao powder

¼ cup coconut nectar

¼ cup maple syrup

1 tsp vanilla bean

2 tsp vanilla extract

Pinch espresso powder

Pinch sea salt

Melt coconut oil by setting jar in bowl of warm water. Once melted, transfer to bowl and add remaining ingredients. Whisk well to combine. Place in serving dish or squirt bottle to serve. Store at room temperature for up to 1 week. If storing in fridge, you will want to place in bowl of warm water to melt and then stir well to recombine.

Hot Fudge Sauce

Makes about 1 cup

Unlike the raw fudge sauce, this cooked version uses heat to create a rich hot fudge sauce like the ones found at your favorite ice cream parlors. It is nearly impossible to find a dairy free fudge sauce on the market today that tastes as good as the original version. However, this recipe makes an identical product that is actually more nutritious and rich in antioxidants.

¾ cup canned light coconut milk

2 Tbsp maple syrup

5 ounces dark chocolate pieces

½ tsp ground espresso

1 tsp vanilla extract

Pinch sea salt

In a saucepan, heat the coconut milk until it starts to simmer. Add in maple syrup, stirring well. Remove from heat and add the pieces of dark chocolate and ground espresso; whisk until melted. Remove from heat and stir in the vanilla extract and sea salt. Store in fridge for up to 3 weeks.

Flaky Pie Crust

Makes 1 – 9" pie crust

Pie crust is extremely hard to perfect. It is so important to have a flaky, buttery and golden brown crust to bring out the flavors of the filling. Because this recipe does not contain sweetener, this crust is suitable for sweet or savory fillings.

½ cup brown rice flour

½ cup tapioca flour

½ cup white rice flour

¼ cup ounces sorghum flour

¼ cup potato starch

1 ½ tsp xanthan gum

½ tsp sea salt

4 oz. Earth Balance soy free spread, COLD

3 oz. palm shortening or coconut oil

3 oz. iced water (approximately)

Place the flours, xanthan gum and sea salt into a large bowl and whisk to combine. Cut in Earth Balance and shortening using a pastry blender or your hands and work the dough until pea size balls form. Add water, adding more if needed, until the dough is dry yet sticky. Form into a disc, wrap in plastic wrap and refrigerate for at least 1 hour.

When ready to use, flour surface with tapioca flour and roll out the dough and fit it into a 9-inch pie pan. Place in freezer for 15 minutes. Bake the pie dough at 400° F for about 25 minutes or until golden brown. Cool before filling.

Whipped Cream

It is amazing that coconut cream makes such a wonderful whipped cream. You no longer have to forego the dessert topping with these homemade whipped cream recipes to make your day extraordinary.

Instructions for all recipes:

Spoon solid cream from the top of coconut milk into a chilled metal mixing bowl, leaving opaque gray liquid behind. Add remaining ingredients and whip with hand mixer until fluffy.

Variations:

Plain Whipped Cream

1 – 14 oz. can full fat coconut milk, refrigerated overnight

3 Tbsp organic powdered sugar

1 Tbsp vanilla extract or to taste

¼ tsp vegan gelatin bloomed for 5 minutes in 1 Tbsp water

Pinch sea salt

Pumpkin Whipped Cream

1 – 14 oz. can full fat coconut milk, refrigerated overnight

½ cup canned pumpkin

¼ tsp pumpkin pie spice

1 Tbsp maple syrup

¼ tsp vegan gelatin bloomed for 5 minutes in 1 Tbsp water

Pinch Himalayan salt

Cocoa Whipped Cream

1 – 14 oz. can full fat coconut milk, refrigerated overnight

¼ cup cocoa powder

¼ tsp espresso powder

1 Tbsp maple syrup

¼ tsp vegan gelatin bloomed for 5 minutes in 1 Tbsp water

Pinch Himalayan salt

Mesquite Chestnut Whip

1 – 14 oz. can full fat coconut milk, refrigerated overnight

¼ cup raw cacao powder

¼ cup pureed chestnuts, chilled

1 Tbsp mesquite powder

¼ tsp espresso powder

2 packets stevia

1 tsp chocolate extract

Pinch sea salt

Spoon solid cream from the top of coconut milk into a chilled metal mixing bowl, leaving opaque gray liquid behind. Add remaining ingredients and whip with hand mixer until fluffy.

Cashew Cream

Makes 3 cups

This recipe is a must have for any dairy free kitchen. Using cashew cream in dishes helps replace cheese and creamy sauces. It also serves as a wonderful condiment for a number of items including tacos, salads, soups, sandwiches and even desserts. A high speed blender is recommended to achieve the ideal creamy and sensuous texture.

1 ½ cups raw cashews
1 ½ cups filtered water
1 tsp lemon juice
¼ tsp sea salt

Blend all ingredients in high speed blender until smooth and creamy. Chill. Store in fridge for up to one week.

DESSERTS

Éclair Cake

Serves 8

My trips to the local Italian bakery were cut short when I was diagnosed with food allergies. When a friend introduced me to her Éclair Cake I knew that I could modify it to meet our needs. And I did! It is wonderful for potlucks and holiday festivities. I hope you find this treat to be a wonderful addition to your repertoire.

Pudding:

3 ¾ cups unsweetened vanilla almond milk, divided

¼ cup organic cornstarch

½ cup organic sugar

Pinch sea salt

3 dropperfuls vanilla flavored liquid stevia

1 ½ tsp vanilla extract

1 Tbsp Earth Balance soy free spread

Combine 3 cups milk, sugar, and salt in a medium saucepan and whisk until incorporated. Whisk together remaining ¾ cup milk and cornstarch until there are no clumps and add to saucepan.

Cook the mixture over medium heat, whisking often, until the pudding begins to thicken and just starts to bubble, about 5 to 6 minutes. Reduce the heat to medium low and switch to a rubber spatula. Stir constantly, scraping the bottom and sides of the pan, until the pudding coats the back of a spoon. Remove from heat and stir in stevia, vanilla and Earth Balance. Pour into a bowl and press a piece of plastic wrap onto pudding to prevent skin from forming. Chill for 2 hours.

RECIPES • DESSERTS

<u>Whipped cream:</u>

2 – 3 oz. cans coconut cream

1 Tbsp organic powdered sugar

1 tsp vanilla

½ tsp unflavored gelatin powder

Chill coconut cream in fridge overnight. Whip all ingredients using a hand mixer until fluffy. Fold into the pudding.

<u>Recipe Instructions:</u>

Place a layer of Sarah's Graham Crackers (see Snacks) in the bottom of a baking dish. Top with a layer of the pudding mixture until about ½" – ¾" thick. Repeat. Finally, add one more layer of Sarah's Graham Crackers and pour ganache (recipe below) over the top. Chill for 6 hours.

<u>Ganache:</u>

½ cup vegan mini chocolate chips

½ cup coconut milk creamer

Pinch sea salt

1 tsp vanilla extract

Combine chocolate chips and creamer in a small saucepan over low heat. Cook until melted, stirring constantly. Remove from heat and stir in sea salt and vanilla.

Cut Out Cookies

Makes approximately 3 dozen cookies

Cut out cookies are a holiday tradition in many homes. Unfortunately, there are few truly tasty recipes that are also allergy friendly, so I devised this recipe for my friend's kids who have multiple food allergies. It was a hit and I am sure it will become a holiday favorite in your household as well.

½ cup white rice flour

½ cup sorghum flour

½ cup brown rice flour

½ cup tapioca flour

½ cup white teff flour

½ cup arrowroot

1 tsp xanthan gum

1 tsp baking powder

½ tsp sea salt

¼ cup vegetable shortening

¼ cup Earth Balance soy free spread

¾ cup organic sugar

Egg replacer for 1 egg

1 Tbsp vanilla extract

1 tsp almond or orange extract

In a large mixing bowl, whisk together the flours, arrowroot, xanthan gum, baking powder, and salt; set aside.

In the bowl of a mixer, beat the shortening, Earth Balance and sugar until smooth. Add the egg replacer, vanilla and almond extracts and beat until blended. On low speed, slowly add the flour mixture and blend until smooth. Pour dough onto a work surface and gently knead until the dough forms a nice ball. Divide the dough into two round discs, wrap them gently in plastic, and refrigerate for 1 hour.

When you are ready to make your cookies, preheat your oven to 375°F and line a cookie sheet with parchment paper. Place one of the discs on a piece of parchment that has been dusted with rice flour. Place plastic wrap over the top of the dough and roll the dough into ¼" thickness. Remove the plastic and cut using cookie-cutters. Place on baking sheet and bake for 10-15 minutes, rotating the tray half way through. Cool on a wire rack and ice (recipe below) if desired.

Icing:

2 cups organic powdered sugar

1 tsp pure vanilla extract

4 to 6 Tbsp orange juice, or more if needed

Mocha Maca Mousse

Serves 6

This is hands-down one of the most incredibly decadent and indulgent recipes in my arsenal. Deep, dark, rich and irresistible. Yum!

½ cup pitted medjool dates, soaked in water for 3-4 hours, and drained

½ cup pure maple syrup

¼ cup brewed espresso or coffee

2 tsp vanilla beans, scraped from pod

3 avocados

¾ cup raw cacao powder

¼ cup coconut butter

2 Tbsp maca powder

Pinch sea salt

¼ cup coconut milk

Place the dates, maple syrup, espresso, and vanilla bean in a food processor and process until smooth. Add the avocado, cacao powder, coconut butter, maca powder, and sea salt and process until creamy. Stop occasionally to scrape down the sides of the bowl with a rubber spatula. Add the coconut milk and process briefly until creamy and thick to your desired texture. Serve chilled or at room temperature.

Pecan Sandies

Makes 3 dozen cookies

Words alone cannot even begin to describe the irresistible taste and texture of these delicious homemade cookies. I can devour a plate of these buttery, melt-in-your-mouth treats. There never seems to be enough of these cookies because they tend to disappear quickly. I enjoy these cookies with a glass of Cashew Milk (see Beverages).

1 cup Earth Balance soy free spread
⅓ cup coconut palm sugar
2 tsp water
2 tsp vanilla extract
2 cups Sarah's All Purpose Flour Blend
1 cup chopped pecans
Organic Powdered Sugar

In a medium bowl, beat Earth Balance and sugar with hand mixer until creamy. Add water and vanilla and mix well. Beat in the flour until just combined. Fold in the pecans and form the dough into a ball. Chill for 4 hours.

Preheat oven to 325°F.

After dough has been chilled, shape dough into 1" balls. Place on cookie sheet and bake for 20 minutes. Remove from pan and roll in organic powdered sugar if desired. Cool on wire rack.

Chocolate Cupcakes

Makes 16 standard size cupcakes

Who doesn't love a moist, rich cupcake? Gluten free baked goods do not have to be dense and un-flavorful. The marvelous taste of these chocolate cupcakes will amaze your guests and are wonderful for that birthday celebration.

Coconut oil cooking spray

1 cup coconut palm sugar

½ cup brown rice flour

½ cup almond flour

¾ cup unsweetened Dutch-process cocoa powder

¼ cup potato starch

¼ cup sweet rice flour

2 tsp baking soda

1 tsp baking powder

¾ tsp sea salt

¼ cup applesauce

Egg replacer for 1 egg

¾ cup warm water

4 oz. unsweetened coconut milk yogurt

2 Tbsp vegetable shortening, red palm oil, or Earth Balance soy free spread

1 tsp vanilla extract

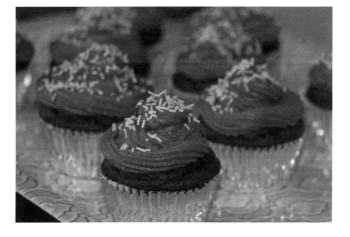

Preheat oven to 350°F. Place baking cups in each muffin pan cavity.

Whisk together the coconut palm sugar, brown rice flour, almond flour, cocoa powder, potato starch, sweet rice flour, baking soda, baking powder, and sea salt in a large bowl. Using a hand mixer, add the applesauce, egg replacer, water, yogurt, shortening and vanilla and blend until smooth. Divide batter between baking cup lined muffin pans. Bake cupcakes for about 20 minutes or until a toothpick comes out clean. Cool on wire racks.

"Buttercream" Frosting

2 squares semisweet bakers chocolate, melted and cooled

1 cup Spectrum butter flavored shortening

1 cup organic powdered sugar

¼ cup raw cacao powder

2 Tbsp unsweetened non-dairy milk

1 Tbsp vanilla extract

Pinch sea salt

Place all ingredients into a mixing bowl and whip with an electric mixer until light and fluffy. Use to frost cupcakes.

Sarah's Famous Chocolate Chippers

Makes 20 - 1 ½" cookies

The best chocolate chip cookie ever! These chocolate chip cookies are the best mix of chewy and crunchy and are thick with bittersweet chocolate morsels studded throughout each irresistible bite.

½ cup superfine brown rice flour

½ cup tapioca starch

½ cup gluten free oat flour

¼ cup millet flour

2 Tbsp organic cornstarch

2 Tbsp potato starch

1 tsp baking soda

½ tsp baking powder

½ tsp sea salt

¼ tsp xanthan gum

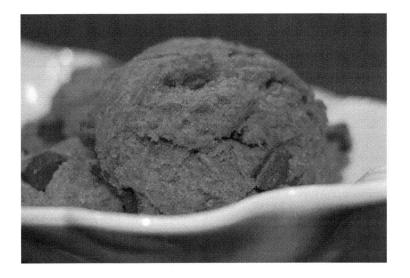

¾ cup coconut palm sugar

½ cup packed organic light brown sugar

½ cup Earth Balance soy free spread

¼ cup coconut oil

¼ cup applesauce

1 Tbsp ground chia mixed with 3 Tbsp warm water

1 tsp vanilla extract

½ tsp vanilla bean

1 bag vegan dark chocolate chunks

½ cup chopped pecans (optional)

Preheat oven to 350°F.

In a large bowl, whisk together the flours, cornstarch, xanthan gum, baking soda, baking powder, and sea salt.

In the bowl of a stand mixer, cream together the sugars, Earth Balance, chia mixture, vanilla extract, and vanilla bean. Turn the mixer on low and slowly add the flour mixture. Stir in the chocolate chips and nuts, if using. Chill dough for 30 minutes.

Scoop dough into 1 ½" balls and place on parchment lined cookie sheet. Bake for 18 to 20 minutes or until edges are golden brown. Cool on wire rack.

Frosted Sugar Pillow Cookies

Makes approximately 30 – 1 ½" cookies

These cookies are for those who prefer soft, pillowy cookies like those you see in the bakery section of the grocery store with the icing and sprinkles. Frosting makes these extra special, however, I personally prefer them unfrosted. I hope you share these with your loved ones as they will quickly become a family favorite.

¾ cup organic sugar

½ cup Earth Balance soy free spread

2 Tbsp vegetable shortening

½ cup unsweetened coconut milk yogurt

2 Tbsp applesauce

2 tsp vanilla extract

½ tsp almond extract

½ cup superfine white rice flour

½ cup superfine brown rice flour

½ cup tapioca flour

½ cup potato starch

¼ cup gluten free oat flour

2 Tbsp sweet rice flour

2 Tbsp organic powdered sugar

1 Tbsp organic cornstarch

1 ½ tsp baking powder

1 tsp baking soda

1 tsp xanthan gum

½ tsp sea salt

In a mixer bowl, cream the sugar, Earth Balance and shortening together until fluffy. Add the yogurt, applesauce, vanilla and almond extract, and beat until combined.

In a medium bowl, whisk together the flours, powdered sugar, cornstarch, baking powder, baking soda, xanthan gum, and sea salt. Gradually add the flour blend to the mixer, running on low and scraping the sides occasionally until fully incorporated. Pour dough out onto a floured surface and form into a disc. Wrap in plastic wrap and chill for 1 hour.

Preheat oven to 400°F.

Roll the dough between parchment paper sheets with a rolling pin to ¼" thickness and cut using desired cookie cutter shape. Place on a cookie sheet and bake for 10 minutes or until edges start to brown. Cool on a wire rack.

<u>Frosting</u>:
½ cup Earth Balance soy free spread, softened
2 cups organic powdered sugar
2 Tbsp plain coconut creamer
1 Tbsp vanilla extract
Pinch sea salt
Natural food coloring, if desired

Whip all ingredients together using a hand mixer. Frost cooled cookies.

Blueberry Lavender Ice Cream

Serves 8

This is by far my most requested recipe. The blueberries make this ice cream vibrant purplish-blue in color, and the delicate floral splash of the lavender simply to die for.

1 can full fat coconut milk

1 cup coconut creamer

½ cup coconut organic sugar

1 dropperful vanilla stevia

1 tsp vanilla extract

1 tsp guar gum

2 cups fresh blueberries

1 Tbsp dried lavender

½ tsp cinnamon

Combine the coconut milk, creamer, sugar, stevia, guar gum and vanilla in blender and run until smooth. Add in blueberries and cinnamon and lightly pulse. Stir in lavender. Keep overnight in fridge for flavors to blend, then pour into ice cream maker and use according to manufacturer's instructions.

Maple Pecan Ice Cream

Serves 8

Who doesn't love an ice cream sundae on a hot summer's day? I know I do! I also like to experiment with the flavor. A whisper of saltiness makes his ice cream addictive. The velvety, smooth texture is thick and rich so just a small amount is enough to satisfy any sweet tooth.

3 cups water

4 pitted dates

¼ cup organic brown sugar

¼ cup maple syrup

4 tsp maple extract

2 packets stevia

½ tsp sea salt

1 tsp sunflower lecithin

1 tsp guar gum

½ cup chopped pecans

Puree all ingredients in a high speed blender until smooth. Pour into ice cream maker and process according to manufacturer instructions. When ice cream is thick, add nuts. If desired, serve topped with Caramel Sauce.

Caramel Sauce

½ cup coconut nectar

½ cup maple syrup

¼ cup coconut creamer

¼ cup Earth Balance soy free spread

½ tsp baking soda

1 tsp vanilla extract

Pinch sea salt

Warm large sauce pan over medium heat, add nectar, maple syrup, creamer and Earth Balance to warm pan. The mixture should bubble gently. Turn heat to medium low and stir continuously. After 10 or so minutes, the mixture will thicken. Remove from heat and whisk in baking soda, whisking for 2 to 3 minutes. Remove from heat, stir in vanilla and sea salt, and cool to room temperature.

Orange Chiffon Pie

Makes 1 nine inch pie

Orange Chiffon Pie is very sacred to me. Thanksgiving has always been my favorite holiday and this pie was served each year because it was my Grandmother's favorite recipe. Her Pumpkin Chiffon Pie was also amazing but the creamy orange flavor of this pie prevails over all other pies. Delightful!

3 egg yolks

¼ tsp sea salt

1 tsp orange zest

3 Tbsp cold orange juice

1 Tbsp lemon juice

¾ cup organic sugar, reserved

4 Tbsp orange or lemon flavored gelatin

½ cup hot orange juice

3 egg whites

¼ tsp cream of tartar

1 baked pie shell (see recipe)

Beat egg yolk with whisk in double boiler. Whisk in sea salt, orange zest, 3 Tbsp cold orange juice, lemon juice and 6 Tbsp of the sugar. Cook over medium heat until mixture thickens and coats the back of a spoon. Stir in ½ cup hot orange juice into the gelatin and stir until gelatin fully dissolved. Cool until set (about an hour).

In another bowl, beat egg whites with cream of tartar until stiff peaks form. Beat in remaining sugar. Next, fold in the cooled custard mixture. Pour filling into baked pie crust and chill for 2 hours or more.

Berry Cobbler

Serves 10

Berry Cobbler is a favorite among my catering clients and I have to admit it is a favorite of mine as well, especially topped with Almond Infused Vegan Whipped Cream. What's not to enjoy about a warm and luxurious bowl of berries and cream?

½ cup brown rice flour

½ cup almond or other whole grain flour

½ cup tapioca flour

2 tsp baking powder

½ tsp salt

4 ounces Earth Balance soy free spread, cut into small pieces

¾ cup cold original coconut creamer, plus more for brushing

¼ tsp ground cinnamon

⅓ cup coconut palm sugar, plus more for sprinkling

3 Tbsp cornstarch

6 cups berries

¼ cup sliced almonds

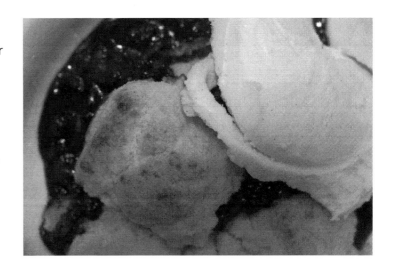

Preheat oven to 375°F.

Pulse flours, baking powder, and salt in a food processor until combined. Add Earth Balance; process until mixture resembles coarse meal. Transfer mixture to a large bowl, and add creamer in a slow, steady stream, mixing with a wooden spoon until dough just comes together.

In a large bowl, whisk together cinnamon, sugar, and cornstarch. Add the berries, tossing gently to coat.

Transfer mixture to a casserole dish. Spoon dough into balls atop the berries, spacing evenly. Brush dough with creamer; sprinkle with sugar and almonds. Bake until berries are bubbling in center and biscuits are golden brown, 45 to 50 minutes. Transfer dish to a wire rack and let cool slightly, about 30 minutes.

Rich Fudgy Brownies

Makes 12 brownies

The name of this recipe says it best. I have been well known to have a mild (or extreme) addiction to chocolate. This recipe was inspired by my grandmother's fondness for brownies. Adding peppermint oil and crushed candy canes make a delightful treat to leave for Santa on Christmas Eve.

½ cup pumpkin puree

½ cup coconut palm sugar

¼ cup powdered sugar

1 tsp baking powder

½ tsp xanthan gum

¼ cup superfine brown rice flour

¼ cup tapioca flour

2 squares bittersweet baking chocolate, melted with ¼ cup coconut oil

2 tsp vanilla extract

1 cup chopped walnuts (if desired)

Preheat oven to 375°F.

In a medium bowl, mix the pumpkin puree, coconut palm sugar and coconut sugar with a hand mixer. Next, beat in baking powder, xanthan gum, brown rice flour, and tapioca flour. With a spatula, fold in melted chocolate blend, vanilla, and walnuts. Bake for 25 minutes or until a toothpick comes out clean.

Baked Chocolate Custard

Makes 6 servings

Rich, delicious and intense in chocolate flavor. I bring this to parties because it is safe to leave out since there are no eggs. The best part is that no one has any idea that this is made with squash. I am confident you will fall in love with this easy to make dessert.

2 cups butternut squash puree

⅓ cup cocoa powder

¼ cup coconut palm sugar

½ cup melted high quality chocolate

¼ cup almond flour

1 tsp baking powder

2 tsp vanilla extract

½ tsp sea salt

¼ cup slivered almonds

Preheat oven to 375 °F degrees.

Place all ingredients except slivered almonds into a high speed blender and blend until smooth. Spoon mixture into greased baking dish. Top with slivered almonds and bake for 30 minutes.

Jam Thumbprint Cookies

Makes 2 dozen cookies

Thumbprint cookies are so pretty and tantalizing. I admire their versatility when it comes to topping options. This recipe uses fruit spread, however nut butter, frosting or cashew cream are also delicious. Kids love to squish their thumbs and fingers into these family favorites.

½ cup Earth Balance coconut spread

¼ cup Spectrum palm shortening

½ cup coconut palm sugar

2 tsp vanilla extract

1 tsp almond extract

½ cup almond meal

⅓ cup tapioca flour

⅓ cup sorghum flour

⅓ cup superfine brown rice flour

¼ cup potato starch

1 tsp xanthan gum

1 jar fruit spread of choice

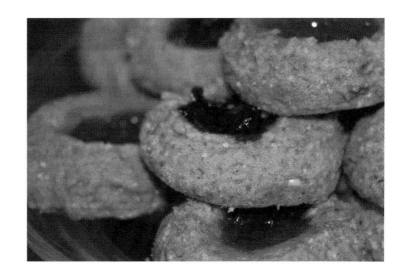

Preheat oven to 350°F. Line a cookie sheet with parchment paper.

Using a hand mixer, beat Earth Balance, shortening, palm sugar and extracts in bowl for 3 minutes, until light and fluffy. Add in remaining cookie ingredients and combine well. Let dough rest for 10 minutes. Roll 1 to 2 Tbsp of dough into a ball (batter will be wet) and place on a parchment-lined cookie sheet. Indent the cookies using your thumb and drop approximately 1 tsp of fruit spread into each indentation. Bake for 15 minutes.

Remove from oven and allow the cookies to sit on baking sheet for 5 minutes. Transfer to a wire rack to continue cooling.

Indian Pudding

Serves 8

Although I did not love this pudding as a child because of the robust molasses flavor, I love it as an adult. As a kid I used to mound whipped cream on top to soften the flavor, but now I enjoy my pudding with a dollop of vanilla vegan whipped coconut cream. My mom says, "There's nothing better on a cold winter day!"

¼ cup quick cook tapioca (pudding aisle)

4 cups non-dairy milk (not rice as the pudding will not set)

3 Tbsp organic cornmeal

½ cup molasses (not blackstrap)

2 Tbsp Earth Balance soy free spread

2 eggs, beaten

6 Tbsp coconut palm sugar

½ tsp sea salt

½ tsp cinnamon

¼ tsp ground ginger

Pinch allspice

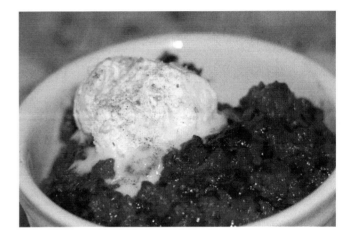

Preheat oven to 350°F.

In a medium saucepan, cook tapioca in milk over medium heat until clear, about 8 minutes. Stir in cornmeal and cook for 15 minutes. Cool to room temperature. When cooled, add the remaining ingredients and whisk well to combine thoroughly. Pour into a greased 1 ½ quart baking dish greased with coconut oil. Bake for 2 hours.

Fruit & Nut Clusters

Makes 12 candies

Making your own candy is easy when you have quality ingredients. These take minutes to prepare and are wonderful. I like to store them in the freezer and eat them frozen.

½ cup creamy roasted almond butter

½ cup maple syrup

1 cup raw slivered almonds

¼ cup dried cherries, chopped (or other dried fruit of choice)

1 cup dark chocolate chips 73% cacao

1 tsp vanilla extract

Pinch flaked sea salt

Combine almond butter and maple syrup in a medium saucepan over low heat. Cook, stirring constantly, until almond butter is melted. Remove from heat and stir in almonds and cherries. Allow mixture to cool a few minutes. Drop the almond mixture by the tablespoonful onto a parchment lined cookie sheet and place in the freezer for 10 minutes.

Meanwhile, melt chocolate in a medium saucepan over lowest heat possible, stirring continuously. Remove from heat and stir in vanilla. Next, remove the almond clusters from freezer and spoon the melted chocolate over each cluster. Sprinkle with sea salt and chill in fridge for at least 20 minutes or until set.

Orange Cranberry Bars

Makes 16 bars

This is certainly not the healthiest dessert, but certainly is one of the tastiest. I bring this bar to picnics because it is heat safe. Rain or shine, these bars are a picnic hit. You will see what I mean when you taste these rays of sunshine.

Crust:

½ cup gluten free oat flour

½ cup sorghum flour

½ cup teff flour

½ cup tapioca flour

Pinch sea salt

¾ cup organic powdered sugar

Pinch sea salt

8 oz. Earth Balance soy free spread, room temperature

2 tsp orange extract

For the filling:

8 oz. fruit juice sweetened orange marmalade

½ cup soaked fruit juice sweetened cranberries

8 oz. vegan plain non-dairy cream cheese, room temperature

For the topping:

¾ cup quick cook gluten free oats

¾ cup sweet rice flour

8 oz. Earth Balance soy free spread, room temperature

¼ cup organic brown sugar

Pinch sea salt

Zest of an orange

Preheat oven to 350 degrees. Prepare a 9x13" pan with nonstick cooking spray and set aside.

For the crust, mix all ingredients together in a bowl until you have ball of dough. Place ball in the prepared pan and flatten, making sure it covers the entire bottom of pan and is about ¼" thick. Bake for 22 minutes or until golden brown. Once crust is removed from oven, let cool for 10 minutes.

While crust is baking prepare topping in the same bowl, mixing all ingredients until it is crumbly.

In a small mixing bowl, mix marmalade and cranberries together. Then spread cream cheese on crust and spoon marmalade mixture over cream cheese. Now sprinkle the cranberries over the marmalade and bake for 20 minutes or until topping is golden brown. Allow to cool before cutting and serving.

Kicked Up Chocolate Ginger Ice Cream

Makes 1 ½ quarts

This ice cream is incredibly deep, dark and luxurious. It pairs sweet and spicy candied ginger with a silky cashew base to charm the palate. I guarantee any chocolate lover will come back for more.

3 ½ cups water

2 cups cashews

1/3 cup cocoa powder

2 Tbsp fresh grated ginger

¼ cup yacon syrup

2 Tbsp coconut palm sugar

2 packets stevia, or 2 dropperfuls chocolate stevia

½ tsp guar gum (can be omitted if eating immediately)

1 tsp vanilla extract

¼ cup candied ginger, chopped

½ cup vegan dark chocolate, chopped

Combine all of the ingredients, except candied ginger and dark chocolate chunks, in a high speed blender. Run on high until completely smooth. Pour into an ice cream maker and freeze according to manufacturer's directions. When finished, mix in the chopped candied ginger and chocolate. Serve immediately or freeze.

SAMPLE MEAL PLAN

HONESTLY GLUTEN FREE & DAIRY FREE

Sunday

Breakfast: Eggless Omelet, half grapefruit

Lunch: Minestrone Soup with Anti-Aging Salad, few Grain Free Crackers

Snack: Banana Honey Molasses Muffin with 12 raw almonds

Supper: Vegatarian Stuffed Peppers, steamed broccoli, roasted carrots

Monday

Breakfast: Dreamy Creamy Orange Shake with greens and vegan protein powder

Lunch: Bistro Chicken Salad made on bed of romaine lettuce, Fall Fruit Salad

Snack: Sarah's Vitality Ball

Supper: Honey Balsamic Chicken, Happy Hempseed Salad

Dessert: Berry Cobbler

Tuesday

Breakfast: Breakfast Brown Rice, fresh apple with cinnamon, plain almond milk yogurt

Lunch: Super Green Chopped Salad, side of Corn Pudding

Snack: Crunchy Chickpea Poppers, 1 medium apple

Supper: Crockpot White Turkey Chili, Celery and Broccoli Salad

Wednesday

Breakfast: Crockpot Steel Cut Oats, Blueberry Breakfast Burger

Lunch: Simple Veggie Burger, Creamy Roasted Red Pepper, Tomato and Artichoke Soup

Snack: Sarah's Favorite Crunchy Protein Bar

Supper: Simple Fish Tacos with Blueberry and Mango Salsa, Curried Carrot and Zucchini Salad,
Roasted Cauliflower with Apple and Dill

Thursday

Breakfast: Vegan Southwest Scramble, side of black beans, Salsa and Guacamole

Lunch: Clam Chowder with Whole Grain Dinner Rolle

Snack: Frozen Mocha Maca Latte

Supper: Stuffed Turkey, Quinoa Stuffing, mashed cauliflower with sauteed spinach and garlic

Friday

Breakfast: Breakfast Stuffed Sweet Potato, 2 sliced kiwi fruit

Lunch: Mike's Vegetable Beef Soup with Anti-Aging Salad

Snack: Graham Crackers with Surprising Chocolate Dip

Supper: Pumpkin Pizza and Unruly Caesar Salad

Dessert: Blueberry Lavender Ice Cream

Saturday

Breakfast: Protein Pancake topped with Cranberry Apple Compote

Lunch: Sunflower Veggie Spread on Fabulous Fiber Bread stuffed with fresh veggies

Snack: Espinaca and Pretzels for dipping

Supper: Ginger Broiled Halibut with Rice Pilaf, roasted asparagus

Dessert: Chocolate Cupcake with Buttercream Frosting

RESOURCES

Skincare, Body Care, and Cleaning Supplies

Ava Anderson Non Toxic: www.nontoxicmomNY.com

Kitchen Essentials

Alter Eco: www.alterecofoods.com

Arrowhead Mills: www.arrowheadmills.com

Artisana: www.artisana.com

Authentic Foods: www.authenticfoods.com

Barry Farms: www.barryfarms.com

Bob's Red Mill: www.bobsredmill.com

Chocolate Decadence: www.chocolatedecadence.com

Coconut Secret: www.coconutsecret.com

Cook's Extracts (gluten free maple extract): www.cooksvanilla.com

Daiya: www.daiya.com

Earth Balance: www.earthbalancenatural.com

Earthbound Farms: www.earthboundfarms.com

Eden Foods: www.edenfoods.com

Ener-G Foods (egg replacer powder, sweet rice flour): www.ener-g.com

Essential Living Foods: www.essentiallivingfoods.com

Frontier Foods: www.frontiercoop.com

Hain: www.hainpurefoods.com

Hodgson Mills: www.hodgsonmills.com

Honeyville: www.honeyvillegrain.com

Kelapo: www.kelapo.com

King Arthur Flour: www.kingarthurflour.com

Lundberg: www.lundberg.com

Maranatha Nut Butters: www.maranatha.com

Navitas: www.navitas.com

Nutiva: www.nutiva.com

Ojio: www.ultimatesuperfoods.com

Once Again Nut Butters: www.onceagain.com

Orgran (egg replacer powder): www.orgran.com

Pascha Chocolate: www.paschachocolate.com

Penzey's Spices: www.penzeys.com

Plainville: www.plainvillefarms.com

Saratoga Peanut Butter: www.yopeanut.com

So Delicious Non-Dairy: www.turtlemountain.com

Spectrum Organics: www.spectrumorganics.com

Stevita: www.stevita.com

Sunfood: www.sunfood.com

Sweet Leaf (liquid stevia extracts): www.sweetleaf.com

Tropical Traditions: www.tropicaltraditions.com

Wellshire Farms: www.wellshirefarms.com

Westbrae: www.westbrae.com

Kitchen Tools and Equipment

Blendtec: www.blendtec.com

Excalibur: www.excalibur.com

Hurom: www.hurom.com

Sur La Table: www.surlatable.com

Vitamix: www.vitamix.com

Williams Sonoma: www.williamssonoma.com

WORKS CITED

Academy of Nutrition and Dietetics. (2014). *Meeting Calcium Recommendations on a Vegan Diet.* Retrieved August 28, 2014, from Vegetarian Nutrition: http://vegetariannutrition.net/docs/Calcium-Vegetarian-Nutrition.pdf

American Heart Association. (2015, July 7). *Inflammation and Heart Disease.* Retrieved July 7, 2015, from American Heart Association: http://www.heart.org/HEARTORG/Conditions/More/MyHeartandStrokeNews/Inflammation-and-Heart-Disease_UCM_432150_Article.jsp

Bauer, J. (n.d.). *Refined Grains: How Food Affects Health.* Retrieved 12 2, 2014, from Joy Bauer: http://www.joybauer.com/food-articles/refined-grains.aspx

Committee, N.S. (2005). *Progress in Autoimmune Diseases Research Report to Congress.* U.S. Department of Health and Human Services.

Dannie, M. (2014, September 13). *Can Foods Prevent Grey Hair?* Retrieved December 12, 2014, from Livestrong: http://www.livestrong.com/article/323815-foods-that-prevent-grey-hair/

Health, O. O. (2012, July 16). *Autoimmune Diseases Fact Sheet.* Retrieved from Women's Health: http://womenshealth.gov/publications/our-publications/fact-sheet/autoimmune-diseases.html#b

Healthwise Staff. (2014, March 12). *C-Reactive Protein (CRP).* Retrieved August 31, 2014, from Web MD: http://www.webmd.com/a-to-z-guides/c-reactive-protein-crp

Ipatenco, S. (2014, January 14). *Which Foods Prevent Free Radicals in Your Body?* Retrieved December 23, 2015, from Livestrong: http://www.livestrong.com/article/500329-what-foods-prevent-free-radicals-in-your-body/

Lehman, S. (2015, Feburary 6). *What Are Enriched and Fortified Foods?* Retrieved February 28, 2015, from About Health: http://nutrition.about.com/od/askyournutritionist/f/enriched.htm

WORKS CITED

McCluskey, C. (2012, July 16). *7 Tips to Naturally Reduce Cellulite*. Retrieved December 23, 2014, from Mind Body Green: http://www.mindbodygreen.com/0-5479/7-Tips-to-Naturally-Reduce-Cellulite.html

Minnesota Department of Health. (n.d.). *Nutrition Facts: Whole Grains*. Retrieved 11 30, 2014, from Minnesota Department of Health: http://www.health.state.mn.us/divs/hpcd/chp/cdrr/nutrition/facts/wholegrains.html

Nagel, R. (2009, May 1). Agave Nectar, the High-Fructose Health Food Fraud. *Townsend Letter*. Retrieved from Agave nectar: the high-fructose health food fraud: http://www.thefreelibrary.com/Agave+nectar%3a+the+high-fructose+health+food+fraud.-a0198715576

Physicians Committee for Responsible Medicine. (n.d.). *Health Concerns about Dairy Products*. Retrieved October 2, 2014, from PCRM.org: http://www.pcrm.org/milk

Reporter, D. M. (2014, July 16). *Arsenic warning over rice milk: Parents warned not to give drink to children because it can contain harmful levels of the chemical*. Retrieved March 2, 2015, from Dailymail.com: http://www.dailymail.co.uk/news/article-2695096/Arsenic-warning-rice-milk-Parents-warned-not-drink-children-contain-harmful-levels-chemical.html

Sears, B. (2005, January 13). *Save yourself from the hidden killer, 'silent inflammation'*. Retrieved September 2, 2014, from Today: http://www.today.com/id/6791181#.VZyEHPlViko

Self Nutrition Data. (n.d.). *Nutritional Effects of Food Processing*. Retrieved December 23, 2014, from Self Nutrition Data: http://nutritiondata.self.com/topics/processing

University of Massachusetts Medical School. (2013, March 28). *You are what you eat -- even the littlest bites: Dietary influences tied to changes in gene expression*. Retrieved 12 22, 2014, from Science Daily: http://www.sciencedaily.com/releases/2013/03/130328125102.htm

Vieira FG1, D. P. (2011, May-June). Factors associated with oxidative stress in women with breast cancer. *Nutr Hospital, 26*(3), 528-536.

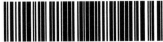

Printed in Great Britain
by Amazon.co.uk, Ltd.,
Marston Gate.